Foundations in Nursing and Health Care

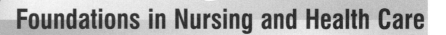

Southampton City College
Learning

Introduction to Sociology for Health Carers

Mark Walsh
Series Editor: Lynne Wigens

SOUTHAMPTON
CITY COLLEGE
LEARNING CENTRE

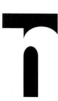

Published in 2004 by:
Nelson Thornes Ltd
Delta Place
27 Bath Road
CHELTENHAM
GL53 7TH
United Kingdom

04 05 06 07 08 / 10 9 8 7 6 5 4 3 2 1

A catalogue record for this book is available from the British Library

ISBN 0 7487 7717 2

Illustrations by Clinton Banbury
Page make-up by Florence Production Ltd.

Printed in Great Britain by Ashford Colour Press

Acknowledgements
Her Majesty's Stationery Office and National Statistics data are subject to Crown Copyright. Crown Copyright material is reproduced with the permission of the controller of HMSO.

Every effort has been made to contact copyright holders and the publishers apologise to anyone whose rights have been overlooked and will be happy to rectify any errors or omissions.

Contents

Preface

The aims of this book are:

- To encourage readers to make connections between health and illness experience, health-care provision and the *social* contexts in which they occur
- To show how sociology and sociological thinking can make a contribution to health-care practitioners' understanding of health and illness experience, their care practice and the organisation of the UK health-care system
- To promote the development and use of a sociological imagination and sociological thinking skills for health-care practice.

This book has been written for students who are beginning pre-registration health care training courses (in nursing, occupational therapy and physiotherapy, for example) and who have little previous experience of studying sociology. As a result, I've tried to make this an accessible, applied introduction to sociology and sociological thinking.

Sociology now features in the basic training courses of all health, social care and welfare professionals. There are very good reasons for this. These will hopefully be obvious by the end of this book. Your understanding of the relevance of sociology for health-care work should gradually be reinforced by each chapter of the book as we take a detailed sociological look at specific health-related topics and build up a knowledge and understanding of what sociology and sociological thinking involve.

The text will avoid adopting a passive 'encyclopedia-of-facts' style of 'information' delivery on the grounds that this makes for a dull book, repeating the approach of many others, and would fail to engage you in sociological thinking in an active, constructive way. I'm aiming to show you how sociological thinking can enhance your development and practice as a health-care worker. As such, it is important for us to consider how sociological thinking and methods can be used constructively and insightfully. Sociology can help us to understand how aspects of 'the social' affect and shape the experience of health and illness as well as our own relationships and practices in the health-care field. In many ways this involves making a case for sociology in terms of its usefulness to you and those you care for and work with. I'll do my best because I think that achieving this is important and worthwhile.

Each chapter includes a number of activity features. These have been included as a way of helping you to apply your learning and develop your sociological thinking skills. It is advisable to have a go at the various activities as they will benefit your learning and understanding of key concepts, skills and issues.

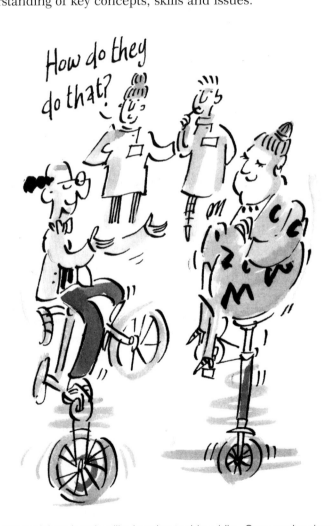

Beginning sociology is rather like learning to ride a bike. Once you've done it, it seems easy, but incredibly difficult to explain to someone else. (Osborne 1999)

Structure of the book

In the first chapter I'll present a basic picture of the origins of sociology and begin to establish its links and relevance to health care. Chapter 2 aims to clarify what is distinctive about the sociological focus and what is involved in 'sociological thinking'. In Chapter 3 we'll apply what has been learnt from the previous chapters by exploring how sociology has been applied to health-care issues.

The next seven chapters (Chapters 4–10) focus on substantive topic areas that link sociology to aspects of the health field. The chapters will consider how sociology has been used to explore and understand how 'the social' enters into and shapes the health-related aspects of each area. I will use examples and make points in each of the chapters to try and persuade you to draw on your knowledge of sociology and use sociological thinking in your health-care practice. Essentially, my argument throughout the book is that developing a 'sociological imagination' and sociological thinking skills will enable you to become a better health-care practitioner. I believe that being able to 'think sociologically' will assist you both personally and professionally in your quest to understand the health field and your place within it.

Mark Walsh

Reference

Osborne, R. (1999) *Introducing Sociology*. Totem Books, London.

Understanding sociology

Learning outcomes

By the end of this chapter you should be able to:

- Describe the origins and evolution of sociology as a discipline
- Describe the distinctive academic focus of sociology
- Consider the relevance of sociology for health-care work.

What is 'sociology'?

Do you have a mental picture of what a 'sociologist' looks like? What are your preconceptions about this particular 'ology'? Reflect on these for a minute or two. However basic, try to express the ideas that you have about what sociologists do and what the subject focuses on. We'll come back to your preconceptions at the end of the chapter. While you may already have some expectations and ideas about sociology and sociologists, this chapter aims to give you a clear understanding of the origins and focus of sociology. I'm also going to begin the process of trying to persuade you that sociology isn't a subject that is only useful to 'sociologists'. I'll argue that it also provides very helpful insights that health carers can apply in their work.

Sociology is a relatively new subject in educational and vocational training institutions. However, it is now possible to begin studying sociology at secondary school, carry on doing so at a further education college and then spend several years getting degrees in it at university. Some people even make a career out of studying and teaching it! This is probably not an attractive idea to most health-care students. In fact, you might even be wondering why it is a part of your health care course at all. In order to appreciate the value of sociology for health care, you first need to gain a basic understanding of the origins, uses and general focus of sociology as a subject or discipline. You will then be in a better position to see its relevance to the health-care field.

The emergence and growth of sociology

The term 'sociology' has Latin and Greek origins and means 'reasoning about the social'. Auguste Compte (1798–1857), a French philosopher who lived through the turbulent social upheavals of the French Revolution of 1789 and the subsequent counter-revolutions, is often given credit for coining the term 'sociology'.

The early 19th century period in which 'sociology' emerged was an era of massive social change. The French Revolution and the longer Industrial Revolution were responsible for reshaping the institutions and 'fabric' of European societies. Social and political relationships were redefined during this period as the power of the Church, the monarchy and the wealthy landed aristocracy was diminished in the face of challenges from utopian social reformers and political revolutionaries. Compte's 'sociology' was an attempt to understand the social changes that were occurring in France during this period and also a grander effort to develop a 'science of society' that could be used to promote progressive social change in the future.

The pioneers of sociology, such as Auguste Compte, established some of the key themes of sociology that remain a part of the discipline today. For example, since the early 19th century sociology has focused on:

- Discovering, and describing the effects of, the dynamics of social change
- Identifying and describing social structures and processes
- Explaining the relationship between the individual and collective 'society'.

The discipline of sociology has evolved and increased in popularity over the last 200 years. It gained greater coherence and much of its academic credibility in the last half of the 20th century. At the beginning of the 21st century, sociology is an established and widely studied academic discipline in its own right. It has a global presence in educational and training institutions, for example, and has generated a substantial body of theoretical and research-based literature on all kinds of specialist sociological topics. As you are now becoming aware, applying sociological theories and methods to areas such as health care has put the subject on the timetables of many different professional training courses. The courses, like your own, in which sociology now features are typically preparing students for 'human services' roles or have a close interest in what has been referred to as 'the human-made world' (Bauman 1990). It is these aspects of the world, the bits that 'bear the imprint of human activity, that would not exist at all but for the actions of human beings' (Bauman 1990), that sociology as a subject is concerned with.

> ## Over to you
>
> - Identify 10 aspects of the world 'that would not exist at all but for the actions of human beings'.
> - Why do you think sociology as a subject might be interested in these aspects of the 'human-made world'?

Sociology and other health-care subjects

Pre-qualifying training courses for health-care practitioners usually cover a range of foundation subject areas. These tend to include the so-called 'natural sciences' (biology, biochemistry, anatomy and physiology, for example) and the 'social sciences' as well as clinical practice and skills inputs. As a result, pre-qualifying courses adopt something of a 'magpie approach' to their knowledge base. They take or borrow theories, concepts and research approaches from the subject areas that are most useful for developing an understanding of the health field.

Sociology is often identified to as a 'social science' discipline within this 'pick and mix' selection. There is a significant debate within and outside of sociology circles about whether it is, or should even seek to be, a 'scientific' discipline. However, despite this, sociology is usually categorised alongside psychology, social policy, anthropology, politics and economics as a 'social science' discipline because, like these other subjects, sociology focuses on human activity and experience. Sociology and psychology are the two social science subjects that are most often drawn on in health-care training courses.

If the social sciences are a new area of study for you, the distinctions between psychology and sociology may be difficult to work out at first. This problem partly occurs because psychology and sociology do 'overlap' at times. It's true that sociologists and psychologists are often interested in exploring similar (sometimes the same) 'human world' topics and issues. However, it's important to note that if sociologists and psychologists do explore the same aspects of the human world they are likely to do so using differing theoretical approaches and by employing research methods in distinctive ways.

What is different about sociology?

A simple way of distinguishing between psychology and sociology is to say that psychology typically focuses on internal aspects of *the individual.* Psychologists generally investigate and develop theories about the factors and processes that affect our internal psychological and emotional processes and behaviours. They're interested in 'personality', 'emotions', 'learning', 'memory' and 'thinking', for example. The individual is, therefore, the main object or focus of psychological research. In contrast, sociology focuses on how aspects of 'the human world' which are external to people affect us *as a collective*. It is more concerned with how external 'social' and 'environmental' factors and processes work together. These are seen to construct and co-ordinate the life chances and experiences of human beings *at a group level* (as, for example, 'nurses', 'pregnant women', 'African–Caribbean men') and within the context of society as a whole. Sociologists are, therefore, interested in 'social class', 'ethnicity' and 'gender' as fields of social relations within the 'human-made world' that affect people at a collective, or group, level.

Sociology is sometimes seen as being concerned with major social problems, such as unemployment, poverty and racism, which affect some people's lives. These aspects of the human world are important and interesting to some people in the sociology community. However, identifying and addressing social problems and the welfare needs of people who experience them is typically the focus of another discipline – social policy. Sociology is one of several disciplines that social policy academics and practitioners draw on. In particular, social policy practitioners are likely to use

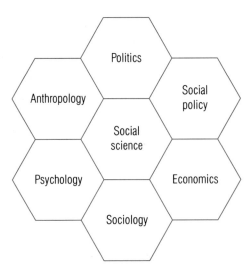

Figure 1.1 *The social sciences are a group of complementary disciplines that focus on organisation, activity and experiences in the human-made world*

sociological thinking and research methods to investigate how and why aspects of the contemporary human world, such as 'social structures', 'social relationships' and 'socio-economic processes', may create the conditions in which these social problems can occur.

The focus of sociology

We've already said that sociology's particular focus is on the 'human-made world'. In doing so it focuses on the relationship between human beings and the 'social' aspects of the human-made world that enter into and shape our collective lives. Sociology therefore focuses on the factors and processes, such as 'gender', 'ethnicity' and 'social class', that shape both our relationships with others and our experience of 'society'. Sociology also focuses on how human lives are socially structured and organised and on the ways in which everyday experiences are made meaningful. Sociology is therefore about both the lives and experiences of people *in* 'the human-made world' (which is also known as 'society') and about the 'social' nature *of* the 'human-made world' itself.

General sociology textbooks, such as Haralambos and Holborn's *Sociology – Themes and Perspectives* (2004), provide a good insight into the aspects of the 'human-made world' that sociology focuses on. They also provide an insight into how academic and professional sociologists have researched and thought about the 'social' aspects of the 'human-made world'. A look at more specialist textbooks, such as those by White (2002), Clarke (2001) and Nettleton (1995), will give you a further insight into how sociology specialists have approached and produced a 'sociological understanding' of the health field. While these books are interesting and useful as a way of gaining an appreciation of the focus of sociology, they do not explain what is special or distinctive about a 'sociological understanding' of health or actively try to get you to produce your own examples of this. However, by the time you have worked through this book, you should be in a position to generate and use 'sociological understanding' in your own health-care practice.

The fundamental goal of sociology, in the first instance, is to generate understanding of the 'human-made world'. As we'll see, there are various ways of approaching this and a number of possibilities of what we can, or ought, to do with this 'sociological understanding' once we've got it. Before we consider these issues, however, we ought to first try to clarify how a 'sociological

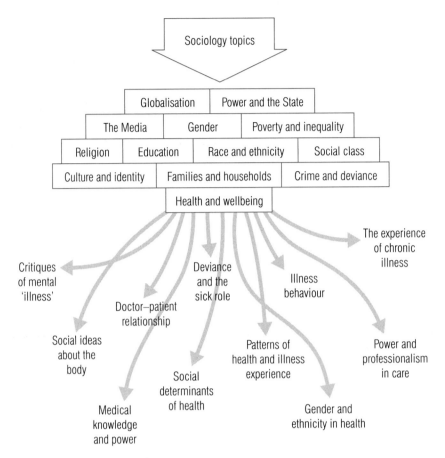

Figure 1.2 *Sociology topics*

understanding' of the human world is different to other forms of understanding. In particular, how does it differ from a 'common-sense understanding' of the world we live in?

Rapid recap

Check your progress so far by working through each of the following questions.

1. Identify when, and explain why, the discipline of sociology first emerged.
2. Explain how sociology differs from psychology.
3. Suggest reasons why the 'human-made world' can be seen as a 'social environment'.

If you have difficulty with more than one of the questions, read through the section again to refresh your understanding before moving on.

References

Bauman, Z. (1990) *Thinking Sociologically*. Blackwell Publishing, Oxford.

Clarke, A. (2001) *The Sociology of Healthcare*. Prentice Hall, Harlow.

Haralambos, M. and Holborn, M. (2004) *Sociology – Themes and Perspectives*, 6th edn. Collins Education, London.

Nettleton, S. (1995) *The Sociology of Health and Illness*. Polity Press, Cambridge.

White, K. (2002) *Sociology of Health and Illness*. Sage, London.

Further reading

Iphofen, R. and Poland, F. (1998) *Sociology in Practice for Health Care Professionals*. Palgrave, Basingstoke.

Jenkins, R. (2002) *Foundations of Sociology – Towards a Better Understanding of the Human World*. Palgrave, Basingstoke.

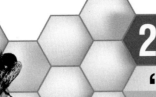

2

'Sociological understanding' and sociological thinking

What is 'sociological thinking'?

Sociology is sometimes criticised for 'stating the obvious' and for claiming to offer insights into the human world that its critics contend are simply 'common sense'. If sociology, as a subject and a way of thinking, is to be useful to you in your health-care work, it should offer a more specific, insightful and powerful way of understanding the health-related aspects of the human world than everyday common sense. But what does it offer? What is distinctive about 'sociological understanding'? And how can it be achieved?

'Sociological understanding' is the result of 'sociological thinking'. In this chapter we're going to consider what it is that people do when they 'think sociologically'. We'll also consider how a 'sociological understanding' of the health-care field is different from (and better than) a common sense understanding of the health-care world.

How does sociological thinking differ from 'common sense'?

Bauman and May (2001) suggest that 'thinking sociologically' is different to 'common sense' thinking because:

● Sociological thinking is based on, and gains its credibility from, the use of *rational, organised, logically structured arguments*.

● Sociological thinking is *evidence-based* and *can be publicly scrutinised* in terms of its appeals to evidence.

● Sociological thinking is based on, and can encompass, *a broad vision* of the social aspects of the human world where common sense does not.

● Sociological thinking always makes sense of the human world by using perspectives that begin with *a collective understanding* of individuals living within 'webs of human interdependency'.

'Sociological thinking' therefore offers a different sort of vision or perspective on the taken-for-granted, familiar aspects of the human world from that offered by 'common sense'. This does not mean that 'common sense' is being criticised for necessarily being wrong or pointless. In fact, 'sociological thinking' and 'common sense thinking' often share a focus on the everyday aspects and meanings of the human world. 'Sociological thinking', however, brings into view a bigger, more detailed and more diverse picture of the human world. It offers us more deliberate, more sensitive and more consciously analytical ways of understanding the human-made world and our experiences within it than common sense.

Sociology and progressive thinking

Bauman and May (2001) argue that 'sociological thinking' is progressive and positive in the sense that it provides us with ways of being more sensitive to and tolerant of human diversity. For example, it makes visible, and makes us aware of, experiences, ways of living, beliefs and values that are different from our own. This makes sociological thinkers question, doubt and often reject arguments about the apparently 'natural', inevitable or unchangeable nature of the human condition, human experiences or the social, political and economic structuring of society.

However, 'sociological thinking' doesn't just enable us to question and criticise the status quo (how things are). It also provides the basis for developing and constructing alternative ways of living, relating and organising society. In doing so, sociological thinking encourages us to engage with and relate to the people around us in more positive, sustaining and mutually supportive ways. In this sense 'sociological thinking' serves a useful moral purpose. The 'sociological understanding' of the world that it can generate provides a potential platform, or resource, that can be used to improve 'the successful management of one's life and the collective management of shared life conditions' (Bauman and May 2001, p. 12).

How can you 'think sociologically'?

If 'sociological thinking' is such a positive, socially progressive thing to do, you'll no doubt want to develop your ability to do it as soon as possible! But what exactly does 'sociological thinking' involve? What are the strategies or steps to gaining a 'sociological understanding' of the human world? The main elements of successful 'sociological thinking' are summarised as key points in the box below. What each of these points involves is then outlined in more detail.

Key points Top tips

- Be sceptical, questioning and critical
- Focus on how 'the social' affects health and health care (and social life generally)
- Contest 'individualist' explanations of health and illness experience
- Think about the 'micro' and the 'macro' levels of society
- Put issues into an historical perspective

Be sceptical, questioning and critical

In some ways 'sociological thinking' involves 'making the familiar strange' by questioning it and by viewing common sense, taken-for-granted assumptions and 'obvious' explanations more sceptically. This is quite an unusual thing to do and can be both attractive to, and difficult for, people who are new to sociology.

Throughout the book we'll look sceptically at how a range of health-related issues are conventionally understood and can be rethought using 'sociological thinking'. Each chapter will provide you with examples of ways in which 'sociological thinking' can be used to generate and argue for new and different ways of understanding health-care issues and experiences. You may find that adopting such a sceptical, questioning approach to the health aspects of the human world is confusing and uncomfortable at times. You'll need to question and reconsider your own often deeply held attitudes, values and beliefs and you may find this unsettling and difficult. You'll also need to confront and find ways of responding to the possibility that in our modern human-made world the success, health and comforts enjoyed by some people may, in fact, be achieved and sustained through the oppression, exploitation and social disadvantage of others.

However, as well as causing you some difficulties at times, developing a more sceptical, open-minded sociological approach to the things that you see and do as a health carer will also be enlightening and rewarding. It will provide you with new ways of seeing and understanding aspects of health and health care that you previously took for granted or never even noticed. It may also offer you an opportunity to think about and adjust your own beliefs and care practices by taking into account the often neglected sociological factors and societal contexts that influence health and illness and our professional responses to it.

Through questioning and being sceptical about 'the social' aspects of the health field you are likely to become engaged in a critique of existing aspects of the human world. This doesn't mean you will necessarily disapprove, or run around saying gloomily that everything is 'wrong' or 'bad'. However, you are likely to adopt a more 'critical' approach by asking questions, such as 'How do they know?' and 'How could it be otherwise?', about what is usually taken for granted. In order to 'think sociologically' in your care practice you'll need to develop systematic doubts about everyday common sense and the taken-for-granted explanations that are part of the contemporary health field.

The use of a critical approach to evidence and theory about the social world gives sociology some of its controversial character because it results in a critique or 'debunking' of everyday understanding. This can challenge the status quo and question or expose established social arrangements and unequal power relations.

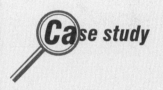

Case study

Louise's clinical placement

Louise is a student nurse. She has just started a clinical placement on an assessment ward for older people with mental health problems. Louise has noticed that the ward staff wake the patients early, at 6.30am, and also ensure that everybody is in bed by 7.30pm before the night shift arrives. When asked why this happens, a charge nurse tells Louise that 'it's common sense to have a regular routine for everyone, especially when a lot of the patients are confused anyway'. He also says that he doesn't think it would be a good idea to 'rock the boat' by changing a system that's so well established on the ward.

Reflective activity

1. What kinds of critical question could Louise ask in response to the charge nurse's explanation?
2. Identify the possible benefits that might result from challenging and changing the status quo that currently exists on the ward.
3. Explain why some members of staff might feel uncomfortable about, and even resentful of, Louise's sceptical, critical questions.

Focus on how 'the social' affects health and health care

The linking of individuals' social behaviours and experiences to a broader social context is one of the distinguishing features of sociological thinking. But what does this 'social context' consist of? Jenkins (2002) describes it as a 'more-than-the sum-of-the-parts' notion that informs sociological thinking in various ways but is particularly evident in the use of two very important sociological concepts.

Society and culture

'Society' is the first of these key concepts. One of the fundamental tenets of sociology is that people live in 'societies'. The term 'society' has a variety of meanings but is typically used to identify the general collectivity to which we belong. 'Societies' are often seen to involve networks of people relating to each other in meaningful ways. The 'meaningful' bit brings in our second key concept – 'culture'. In various ways 'culture' is seen as something that is essential to, and an inevitable part of, any society. It is a concept that holds notions of shared attitudes, values and beliefs and characteristic ways of life. In sociological terms, culture is what binds people together as a collectivity in a society. It is a thing that we share and a 'more-than-the sum-of-the-parts' aspect of the human world that enables us to make human activities and relationships 'meaningful'.

Sensitivity to culture is an important feature of 'sociological thinking' because:

- It helps us to distinguish between the social and natural aspects of human life
- It enables us to identify and acknowledge the existence of social diversity within a society and between different societies
- It allows us to challenge the notion that some social groups and ways of life are 'superior' to others.

A sensitivity to culture and cultural difference allows us to identify, accommodate and respond respectfully to the culturally specific forms that societies and social behaviours take. One consequence of this for health-care workers is that we need to develop and apply an awareness of **culturally diverse** ways of help-seeking and illness behaviour in order to meet the needs of all service users in a culturally diverse population.

The sociological concept of 'cultural relativity' is often used within the health and welfare fields to question the idea that some ways of life are 'better' than others. It also helps to dispel

⚷ Keywords

Cultural diversity
The co-existence of people who have differing cultural heritages and ways of life. The UK is now a culturally diverse country.

◐─┬ Keywords

Ethnocentrism

The situation where the cultural practices or heritage of one group of people are evaluated negatively by an individual (or group) who assumes that their own cultural standards are 'normal' or best. Health-care workers should avoid ethnocentrism because it fails to take cultural difference and diversity into account in a non-judgemental way.

'**ethnocentrism**' or the assumption that one's own culture and society are somehow 'superior' to others. As a result health and welfare workers generally accept the need to avoid making culturally biased (or ethnocentric) judgements about other people. However, applying the concept of 'cultural relativity' can be difficult when it clashes with other strongly held care values. For example, practices such as female genital mutilation and 'forced' marriage are culturally acceptable in some non-Western societies. As individuals, many British health-care workers would, however, find them unacceptable. As health-care workers you might like to consider whether it is possible to reconcile the concept of 'cultural relativity' with Western care values of 'informed consent', 'freedom of choice' and 'protection from harm' in such circumstances.

Fields of social relations

Within sociology, human social relationships and health experiences are generally understood as occurring within 'fields of social relations'. This is another 'more-than-the-sum-of-the-parts' way of thinking about the relationships we have with others. At an individual level, people interact and relate to each other in a myriad of everyday situations, seemingly as individuals. However, thinking sociologically, we would have to argue that 'gender', 'social class' and 'ethnicity' are social factors that affect our collective experiences and shape our behaviour so that we conform to expected social roles.

For example, the constantly developing field of gender relations determines how we become 'masculine' or 'feminine' and think about 'men' and 'women'. This in turn affects the kinds of roles, relationships and behaviours we expect of, and allow, people to perform as gendered subjects. In this sense, as a 'man' or a 'woman' you can't just do what you want or be who you want to be in the human world. Gender structures and processes exist beyond the individual level and act on us collectively to determine what it is possible for us to do and be like as 'men' and 'women'. Therefore we enter into and take part in any social interaction as a gendered human being as well as an individual because of this 'field of social relations'.

Over to you

- Make a list of the ways in which you learnt the social norms associated with your gender.
- How might gender expectations affect the way that service users respond to male and female health-care workers?

⚷ Keywords

Social institution

Regular, organised patterns of social behaviour that exist as a feature of the social world beyond the level of the individual. Hospitals, the family and social class are examples of social institutions that organise specific, comparatively long-lasting patterns of social behaviour.

⚷ Keywords

Individualist explanations

These locate the causes of social action and social experience within the individual. They tend to see personal decisions, lifestyle and behaviour choices as the main factors affecting our health experience. They ignore the influence of broader social structures and processes.

Social structures and institutions

Sociological approaches to the human world generally see 'society' as being structured and organised through '**social institutions**'. These refer to the ways in which regular, collective patterns of social behaviour are structured and organised to provide a framework for our lives. For example, in Western (including British) societies a range of shared 'social' experiences and activities, including raising children, treating illness and disease and developing knowledge and skills occur within 'social institutions'. We call these social institutions 'the family', 'the health-care system' and 'the education system'. They are contemporary society's way of arranging how best to carry out these shared social tasks. They are also seen as evidence of the existence of a 'society' because they illustrate a collective focus and demonstrate that the human-made world is organised around shared arrangements for meeting collective social needs.

Contest individualist explanations of health and illness experience

'Sociological thinking' involves contesting taken-for-granted concepts, theories and issues. In particular, because of its focus on the influence and impact of 'the social' aspects of the human world, sociological thinking questions and contests the contemporary trend towards '**individualist explanations**' in the health-care field. Individualist explanations of health experience and life chances are now a standard feature of 'pop psychology' and have become a staple of daytime television shows and the self-improvement industry. These types of explanation gain some of their authority and credibility from the way that the mass media present them as unproblematic 'truths'. In doing so they typically refer to 'scientific research' and use a medical model approach to health (see pp. 36–41) to justify the 'truth' claim. The outcome is that poor health experience is seen to result from the failings, inadequacies, imperfections, poor choices and bad decisions of people as individuals. This sort of individualist logic is now established as a ubiquitous form of 'common sense'. However, our sceptical 'sociological thinking' approach should tell us that it is wrong and needs to be contested.

> ## Over to you
>
> - Suggest how the current social trend towards increasing obesity in children might be explained in an individualist way.
> - On what grounds can individualist explanations of childhood obesity be criticised?

Individualist explanations of health and illness experience are rejected by sociological thinkers on the grounds that they are largely ill-informed, often victim-blaming and typically locate the 'causes' of a person's health problems or difficulties in either their personal behaviour, their individual choices ('lifestyle') or their lack of knowledge and understanding. In doing so, individualist explanations ignore the possibility that powerful social structures and processes influence health experience and at the very least impose pressures, constraints and limits on what we can and can't do to determine our health, well-being and general life chances.

Individualist explanations are contrary to sociological thinking because they isolate people, as individuals, from the social contexts and the 'webs of human interdependency', or relationship networks, in which we all live. They imply, incorrectly, that an individual can somehow live apart from, and avoid, the influence of a wider social context. They also suggest that an individual's personal destiny and life chances are wholly within their personal control. Sociological thinking tells us that these claims are incorrect.

Health and illness experiences can't be understood as the randomly distributed consequences of 'luck'. Some people are much more likely to experience ill health than others because of the way that 'social' aspects of the human world enter into, shape and impact on their lives (see Chapters 5, 6 and 7 for examples). Similarly, 'good health' doesn't simply result from freely chosen behaviour and lifestyle options. It is an individualist myth that 'health' is achievable simply by exercising personal responsibility and informed judgement. Instead, the social structures, processes and material circumstances that constitute (make up) the human world act upon people, or at least restrict their opportunities to act 'freely', by organising, shaping and even determining the possibilities of their health and illness experience. Sociologically, health and illness experiences must be analysed and explained in relation to the culturally and historically specific, and socially structured, human world in which they occur.

Think about the 'micro' and the 'macro' levels of society

Sociology focuses on both human social behaviour and on the social structures and processes that constitute the human world. In this way 'sociological thinking' requires us to consider the social aspects of the human world at '**micro**' and '**macro**' levels. We need to try and understand both the fine, micro-level details of people's lives (How do people live? What values and beliefs guide social relationships? How do people relate to each other?) and the general, macro-level social contexts in which we all live (How is social life

○━┓ Keywords

'Macro' sociology
Focuses on the large, usually structural aspects of the way that society is organised.

'Micro' sociology
Focuses on the smaller-scale, more detailed aspects of human social behaviour and social processes that operate within society.

organised? What function do the different social institutions perform for society and the individual? How does social class affect our life chances?).

Asking 'micro' sociological questions

Sociological thinkers may focus on the social aspects of the health field at a micro level by asking and exploring basic questions such as:

- What's happening?
- Why?
- What are the consequences?
- How do you know?
- How could it be otherwise?

The processes of thinking sociologically and investigating micro social aspects of the health field involve using a combination of theoretical and research methods. These are discussed in more detail in Chapter 3.

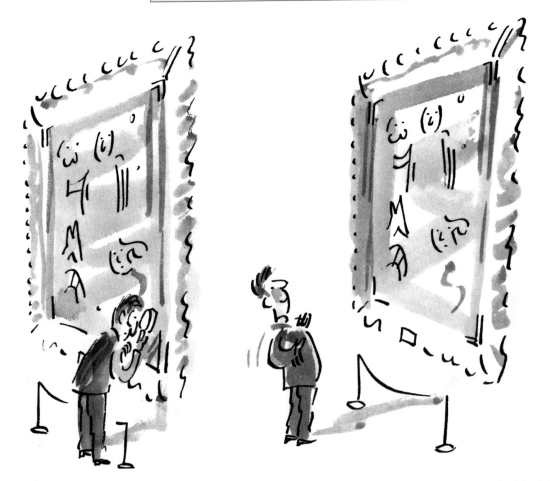

Micro sociology focuses on the detail of social life

Macro sociology is about the big picture

This dual focus – looking at different levels of 'society' – can easily be found in the sociological literature on health and illness. For example, researchers have studied the health aspects of the human world at a micro level by focusing on issues such as doctor–patient relationships and the process of being officially labelled as 'sick'. This form of sociology, in which social roles, interactions and belief systems are seen as key features of social processes and a basis for social relationships, is sometimes referred to as 'micro' sociology. In contrast, so-called 'macro' sociology focuses on the big, often structural, aspects of the health field.

Macro-level sociological thinking involves analysing human social behaviours and the social organisation of the human world in the context of social structure. In doing so, you might, for example, ask the question 'What is it about the way our society is organised as a whole that would explain the existence of poverty?'. An awareness of, and sensitivity to, the presence and influence of social structures is a significant part of thinking sociologically about health and illness experience. For example, is health and illness experience related, somehow, to the structuring of society in terms of class, gender or ethnicity? If so, how does this manifest itself?

Develop a sense of history

Your 'sociological thinking' should, ideally, have an historical backdrop to it. It's important to consider how a person's experiences, or the ways that society is structured and organised, are located in history. For example, present day health-care roles and responsibilities have evolved over time and need to be understood within an historical framework in order to appreciate their significance. You should also realise that a sense of history can always be found in, and is inevitably a part of, all human biographies. As a result, a sociological understanding of a patient's or client's personal biography needs to locate the person's experiences and behaviour historically whilst also noting how this intersects with the social structures and circumstances in which they live.

How can a sense of history help?

- The historical component of the sociological imagination helps us to analyse how 'society' got to be the way it is and to understand how attitudes and behaviours change over time. It enables us to make comparative analyses of different issues.

- An historical awareness helps us to make sense of the ways that society is developing and is organised. It is often possible to understand the present as an evolution of – and sometimes a return to – the past.

- An understanding of history (and culture) enables social phenomena to be located in time (and situated in culture). This enriches our sociological understanding of the world because it allows us to break free from the strait-jacket of thinking only in terms of the society we know in the here and now. Sociologically we need to see society and patterns of social behaviour as a consequence of history and culture.

Developing and using your 'sociological imagination'

The elements of 'sociological thinking' that have just been outlined are well known to academic and professional sociologists and to the many other people who use sociological approaches in their work and personal lives. Many of these people would recognise the things that I have described as features of what is otherwise called 'the sociological imagination'. The idea of a 'sociological imagination' that provides the foundation for, or perhaps an orientation to, 'thinking sociologically' was first developed and expressed by C. Wright Mills, an American sociologist, in 1958. The purpose of the 'sociological imagination' for Mills (1958) was to enable us to understand our 'private troubles' in terms of 'public issues'. That is, Mills believed that many apparently personal experiences that people have, such as unemployment and ill health, can be best understood in the context of wider social forces. For example, unemployment and ill health need to be considered as a consequence of the ways that society is structured and organised and in terms of individual choices and behaviour.

Being a *reflexive* practitioner

Leading on from the idea of the sociological imagination is the suggestion that health-care workers who are able to think sociologically should try to be reflexive practitioners (White and Stancombe 2003). This involves trying to make sociological sense of health-care practices and settings by 'looking outwards' at the way in which society is organised as a whole and in terms of the social groups to which services users belong, as well as 'looking inwards' through personal reflection.

Being reflexive involves considering your own place in the social world, not as an isolated and asocial individual but as someone who both contributes to, and is affected by, the 'greater-than-the-sum-of-the-parts' aspects of the human world. You contribute to the human-made aspects of world via your membership of different social groups and through participating in collective activities. However, your particular experiences of, and responses to, the social world also play a part in constructing and maintaining it. So, your experience of being a health-care worker is partly determined by the social role, status and expectations we presently apply to health-care workers. But it will also vary according to what age, gender, ethnicity, sexual orientation, nationality and social class background you happen to be. As a reflexive practitioner you should be able to look 'outwards' as well as 'inwards' to understand how your own experiences, and those of your colleagues and service users, are historically located and socially situated. In doing so you will be 'thinking sociologically' and will be able to generate your own sociological understandings of the health-care field.

Reflective activity

Using your knowledge and understanding of the main points in the chapter, reflect on the possible ways that 'sociological thinking' and a 'sociological imagination' could improve a health-care worker's ability to provide holistic care for service users.

Rapid recap

Check your progress so far by working through each of the following questions.

1. What is the difference between 'micro' and 'macro' sociology?
2. Identify three features or characteristics of 'sociological thinking'.
3. Explain why sociological thinkers tend to reject individualist explanations of health and illness experience.

If you have difficulty with more than one of the questions, read through the section again to refresh your understanding before moving on.

References

Bauman, Z. and May, T. (2001) *Thinking Sociologically*. Blackwell, Oxford.

Jenkins, R. (2002) *Foundations of Sociology*. Palgrave Macmillan, Basingstoke.

Mills, C. W. (1958) *The Sociological Imagination*. Oxford University Press, New York.

White, S. and Stancombe, J. (2003) *Clinical Judgement in the Health and Welfare Professions*. Open University Press, Maidenhead.

Further reading

White, S. and Stancombe, J. (2003) *Clinical Judgement in the Health and Welfare Professions*. Open University Press, Maidenhead.

3

Sociological approaches to health-care issues

Learning outcomes

By the end of this chapter you should be able to:

- Identify the main features of the positivistic and naturalistic approaches to sociological thinking and theorising

- Explain how sociological approaches can be used to make sense of health-care issues and experiences.

How can we approach health care sociologically?

In the previous chapter we considered what 'sociological thinking' entailed. This involved trying to pin down the core elements of a specifically 'sociological' way of thinking about health issues. To recap, briefly, we said that to 'think sociologically' it is necessary to:

- Be sceptical, questioning and critical
- Focus on how 'the social' affects health and health care
- Contest individualist explanations of health and illness experience
- Think about the 'micro' and the 'macro' levels of society
- Develop a sense of history.

In this chapter we're going to address the question 'How can we *approach* health care sociologically?' The approach part of this sentence is the key issue for us in this chapter. We are now looking for ways of bringing our 'sociological thinking' to bear on health-care issues and on our experiences as health carers.

Unlike disciplines such as physics, mathematics or biology, for example, sociology doesn't have a single method, or even many settled theories, for approaching the social aspects of health care. It would be easier and more reassuring if we were able to use a single approach to make definitive sociological sense of health and health care. Instead we need to be aware of a variety of theoretical approaches and perspectives. Before we consider the kinds of approach and perspectives that are used within sociology we need to come to terms with the slightly scary idea of 'theorising'.

Keywords

Theory
A set of ideas that can be used to explain something. Theories are often based on abstract knowledge or reasoning.

Theorising

Every academic discipline needs and makes use of **theories**. I am a bit reluctant to introduce the term 'theory' because it has such bad connotations. Typically, theories are seen as 'dull', 'complicated' and 'impractical' things that have very little to do with everyday life. 'Theories' are what 'scientists' and 'professors' develop in moments of super-brained inspiration, aren't they? I'm happy to say that this isn't the case as far as much 'sociological' theorising is concerned.

When we 'theorise' about the social aspects of health care we are attempting to make sense of and explain some aspect of it. For example, we would need to theorise in order to explain why people with manual jobs tend to die at an earlier age than their non-manual contemporaries (see pp. 57–59). We would also need to theorise in order to explain the impact that a chronic health problem can have on a person's quality of life (see p. 104 for examples of this). 'Theorising' helps us to give meaning to 'facts' and to make sense of our experiences. It provides us with reasons and explanations. You probably 'theorise' many times a day without even realising. It doesn't necessarily give you a headache but it does ensure that you are not too confused about what's going on in the world!

Thinking about 'reality'

In order to approach health-care issues sociologically, the first point we need to consider is how, in theory, can we know 'reality'? How can we know what's 'true' and 'really' happening in the health field? This is a philosophical issue but one that all sociological thinkers have to address. The question seems complicated but fortunately most sociological thinkers respond with one of two general answers:

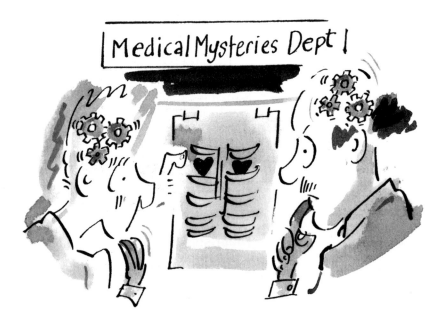

'Theorising' is a common, but often subconscious, activity in health care

- 'By collecting empirical evidence (or "observable facts") about a social reality that exists objectively "out there"'. This is called a *positivistic* approach to social reality.
- 'There is no simple, singular, pre-existing social reality but an infinite range of possible realities constructed by people attributing meaning to their experiences.' This is called a *naturalistic* approach to social reality.

The positivistic and the naturalistic approaches are distinguished by the contrasting **epistemological** stances that they take, that is, by how they claim to know the social world.

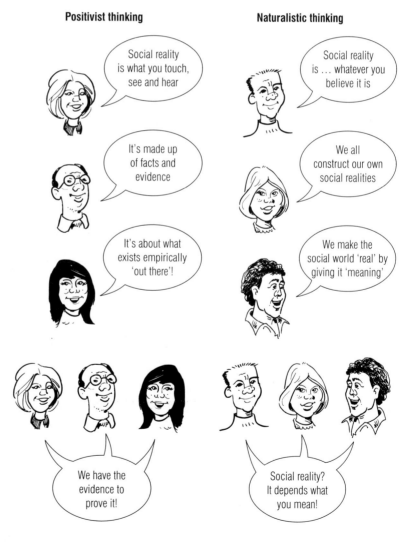

Positivist thinking

Social reality is what you touch, see and hear

It's made up of facts and evidence

It's about what exists empirically 'out there'!

We have the evidence to prove it!

Naturalistic thinking

Social reality is ... whatever you believe it is

We all construct our own social realities

We make the social world 'real' by giving it 'meaning'

Social reality? It depends what you mean!

Figure 3.1 *Thinking about social reality*

Positivistic or 'scientific' approaches

The positivist approach to the social world is sometimes referred to as the 'scientific' or a 'hard' social science approach. Positivists view sociology as a scientific discipline that is similar to the 'natural' sciences (chemistry, physics, biology). They try to emulate the natural sciences by using 'scientific' research methods to investigate the social aspects of health. The goal of positivistic or 'scientific' sociology is to reveal the 'true facts' about society. Ultimately 'scientific' sociology aims to develop strong, empirical 'laws' or statements of generalisable fact about the social world. However, the sociological equivalent of a natural science 'law', such as 'water always boils at 100°C', is very rare and some would say impossible to achieve.

Positivist assumptions

Positivists claim that:

- It is possible to discover and measure 'true facts' about the world
- The methods used to study the physical world can be modified and used to study the social world
- Only 'knowledge' gained through *observed experience* is valid and 'scientific'
- Sociological research that is carried out in a controlled and rigorous way enables scientific 'truths' to be discovered
- Sociological thinkers can, and should, avoid letting their personal biases and interests influence their 'scientific' approach to understanding 'society'

Academic and professional sociologists who accept the basic assumptions of positivism tend to investigate health issues using research tools such as questionnaires, structured interviews and observation checklists because these allow them to collect 'facts' in a controlled way. Additionally, sociologists using a positivist approach typically try to test and observe relationships between 'variables'. Natural or physical variables are the characteristics of entities that can be physically manipulated, such as the heat or volume of a substance. For example, the volume of alcohol that a person is able to consume before becoming unconscious is a variable that is related, in part, to the person's body mass. Larger, heavier people can generally consume more alcohol than smaller, lighter people because of their greater body mass. Social variables are attributes that are assigned to people and that occur in different levels, strengths or amounts within the population. For example, 'marital status' is a social variable that varies in terms of whether a person is single, married or divorced. Other examples of social variables include ethnicity, gender and social class.

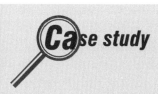

Ali's theory

Ali Shah is an occupational therapy (OT) student. He has some previous experience working as an OT assistant in a social services team. During his time as an OT assistant Ali worked with a large number of people who had acquired physical and sensory disabilities through accidents. Ali became interested in the reasons why some people quickly adapted to, and seemed able to cope with, their acquired disabilities while others took a long time to do so. Ali has a theory about this that he would like to investigate for his dissertation. He thinks that people are more likely to adapt to, and cope with, an acquired disability if they establish a strong, positive and trusting bond with an occupational therapist soon after their accident.

Reflective activity

1. Describe how Ali Shah has 'theorised' the situation described in the case study.
2. Does Ali's thinking suggest that he is taking a positivist approach to this situation? Explain how.
3. Suggest research methods that Ali could use to obtain 'facts' on the issue he's interested in.

Naturalistic or 'interpretative' approaches

Naturalistic approaches to the social world were partly developed out of criticisms of some of the claims and weaknesses of the positivist approach. They are sometimes referred to as 'soft' social science. People who use a naturalistic or 'interpretative' approach to the social world tend to view sociology as a qualitatively different type of discipline from the natural sciences. In sociological research related to health care a naturalistic approach is most likely to be used by members of non-medical disciplines, such as social workers, nurses and occupational therapists, who want to understand the experiences of the individuals and groups that they study from an 'insider's' perspective.

Academic and professional sociologists who adopt a naturalistic approach tend to say that they are 'scientific' to the extent that they carefully select their research problems and investigate them using a systematic research process. However, they would not apply the same 'scientific' criteria or standards to analyse their data, arrive at conclusions or make judgements about social 'reality'. The simple reason for this is that people who use a naturalistic approach believe that it is not possible to apply 'scientific' standards and expectations to the social world because social phenomena are less predictable and uniform than chemical elements or biological processes. Naturalistic sociologists are interested in the *real meaning* of human behaviour and relationships. As a result, they tend to use data collection methods such as participant observation and unstructured in-depth interviews, which allow them to gain access to a wide variety of non-numerical, qualitative data.

Naturalistic sociology tends to focus in detail on specific groups of people, specific social processes or particular social events or situations at a micro-level in the health field. The naturalistic approach is not concerned with trying to discover scientific 'truths' or to establish causal relationships. Instead, naturalistic approaches are based on the idea that human beings are continuously creating their own forms of social knowledge and understanding. As a result no fixed, objective reality exists independently of our culture, values and experience. 'Reality' is therefore a '**social construction**' that is assembled as people interact within a particular context. The human world, and the health field within it, therefore contains multiple realities rather than one single objective social reality. Consequently people who use a naturalistic approach in their sociological thinking try to become aware of, and appreciate how, particular individuals or groups of people view and experience their human world.

⌐ *Keywords*

Social construction
A phenomenon that has been created or developed through social processes rather than being a natural occurrence.

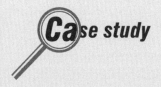

Bryony's project

Bryony Williams is a recently qualified midwife. She has a strong interest in improving the quality of midwifery and obstetric care for women from minority ethnic groups in her local area. Bryony and the midwifery services manager are both aware that ethnic minority women are significantly under-represented as users of local health services generally and midwifery services in particular. However, they don't know why nor have any information on what this group of women want or need from the midwifery team.

ₐₗₗₑₐ**Reflective activity**

1. Explain why a naturalistic approach might be suitable for understanding the midwifery needs of ethnic minority women in this situation.
2. What data collection methods could Bryony use to obtain sociological data on this issue?
3. Explain why Bryony needs to obtain 'insider' data on attitudes, beliefs and cultural practices with regard to childbirth in order to ensure that midwifery services are appropriate to this section of the local population.

ₐₗₗₑₐ**Reflective activity**

When you are developing your own sociological understanding of the human world, reflect on the assumptions you are making. Are you thinking in a positivistic or naturalistic way? Think about both the benefits and the possible limitations of using a particular approach.

Sociological approaches to . . . what?

> In contrast to disciplines such as biology and psychology, which focus on health at the individual level, sociology examines the social dimensions of health, illness and health care.
>
> Daykin 2001

So, now you know how to 'think sociologically' and you can take a considered epistemological stance in your sociological approach to health care. But which aspects of the health field might you want to look at sociologically? What are the 'social dimensions of health, illness and health care' that Daykin (2001) refers to? Again, we have a two-part answer. Sociological approaches to health care tend to focus on:

- How social structures affect health and illness experiences
- How the social actions of individuals and groups play a part in the health field.

Approaching the health field in terms of 'structure' and 'action' takes us back to looking at macro-level structural phenomena or micro-level social actions and processes (see p. 15 for earlier discussion).

Macro-level structural approaches

Structural approaches to the health field involve trying to identify the ways that social structures within society have a determining impact on human health and well-being. Sociologists who are interested in structural issues tend to look at the patterns of health and illness experience at a whole society level. For example, they may be interested in the health and illness experience of whole social classes of people or of men and women as separate social groups. In doing this kind of macro-level sociology academics and researchers are saying that society is differentiated or structured in terms of 'social class' and 'gender' and that class and gender structures have an important impact on people's lives.

Sociological thinking that employs a structural approach tends to view the individual in society as relatively powerless to influence their destiny, health experience or life chances. In an important sense, structural approaches see our lives as powerfully influenced and determined by our place in, and relationship to, social structure. In effect, we're not free to choose how we live or experience the world. Social structures place limits on this and shape the possibilities of our lives. An alternative to this type of **deterministic** structural approach is the social action approach to health and illness.

Keywords

Determinism
The notion that events or situations are predestined because of the existence of other powerful structures or forces.

> ## Over to you
>
> Identify examples of 'structural' forces in society that shape and affect your personal life and your work as a health-care worker.

Micro-level social action approaches

Social action approaches focus on the experiences, social behaviours and everyday lives of individuals and groups in society rather than on the way that social structures affect health and illness experience. For example, sociologists who use social action perspectives investigate and theorise about both the micro-level behaviours of people and the social processes that occur in care settings.

The social action approach is based on the idea that people are relatively free to influence their social experiences and life chances and also play an important part in constructing the social institutions that are a feature of everyday life. This means that macro-level social forces (like social class) are seen as less powerful and deterministic than in the structural approach. According to social action theorists, people have more power, or **agency**, to influence and shape their own lives and destiny than structural perspectives suggest.

Keywords

Agency
The ability people have to act or make decisions either individually or collectively.

Social action approaches argue that people create or construct their social experiences through the cultural meanings that they develop and apply in different social situations. Therefore, individual behaviours and the way of life of different groups in society need to be explored and understood in terms of the specific cultural meanings that group members attribute to them. This sociological point is important for health-care workers who are required to work with a culturally diverse range of people. In a culturally diverse society, a service user's health problems can only be understood by appreciating their cultural perspective and way of life. A health-care worker who is not culturally sensitive and assumes that everyone views 'health' and 'illness', and experiences life, in the same way will fail to identify why a person has health problems and what can be done (appropriately) to help them overcome them.

> ## Over to you
>
> Identify ways in which you believe people can use 'social agency' to influence their chances of achieving and maintaining good 'health'.

Postmodernism

Recent developments in sociological theory have tended to question the forms of thinking that we've just reviewed and that 'traditional' sociology is based on. Postmodernism is a prominent example of this.

One of the key characteristics of postmodernism is its rejection of attempts to devise or present single, all-encompassing explanations of the social world. These all-encompassing theories are often referred to as 'grand narratives'. Examples include Marxist social theories, which claim that social class relations are the key factor that can lead us to the 'Truth' about the organisation and operation of society.

Postmodern social thinkers, on the other hand, tend to adopt a more relativist, subjective approach to the social world. As a result, postmodernism sees the role of sociological thinking as the recognition and acceptance of the rich diversity of beliefs, experiences and perspectives that exist in society. Postmodernists claim that the contemporary social world is characterised by disintegration, uncertainty, eclecticism, cultural democratisation and the questioning of 'expert' knowledge and authority. Postmodernist social thinkers argue that this shift away from accepting 'certainty' towards 'relativism' should be celebrated because it allows us to rethink outdated explanations and approaches to the social world and alerts us to new possibilities for social organisation and activity.

Traditionally, the sociological and other physical and social science theories employed by health-care practitioners have tended to be based on a number of 'universalist' ideas. That is, there has been an acceptance that human beings have universal 'needs', that people have similar health experiences at particular life stages and that we share 'health' goals. Postmodernism is quite effective, however, in drawing attention to the possibility that these 'universal' assumptions are now inadequate. For example, postmodernist thinkers are likely to argue that traditional social and physical science disciplines overlook the particular dimensions of 'need' that are significant for particular individuals and cultural groups. Postmodernism is effective in pointing out that, as health-care practitioners, we may be working with distorted or 'blunt' notions of social identity and human 'need'. In this way it has contributed to a concern with identity and the cultural aspects of health experience as well as raising the visibility and significance of marginalised social groups and their health concerns.

Despite the possibilities that postmodernism offers for the critique and rethinking of our 'traditional' sociological understanding of health-care practice and experience, it has always aroused considerable controversy within the sociology and health-care communities. One of the main criticisms of postmodernism as an approach to sociological thinking is that it lacks a political dimension. That is, it is useful as a way of critiquing or 'deconstructing' other ideas and theories – it is a good way of 'clearing the ground' – but it doesn't actually lead us towards any particular social goal. Postmodernism rejects the idea of social 'evolution' and 'progress' through increasing rational understanding of the social world. It seems to be apolitical in this sense and to ignore the need for social transformation. This can infuriate sociological thinkers who point to the existence of social inequalities and their impact on people's lives and believe that sociological data can inform social and health-care policies that may make the social world a more equitable and equal place.

Contemporary standpoint perspectives

The feminist and anti-racist movements have developed new 'ways of seeing' society and of understanding health experiences that fall outside of the traditional structure/action typology. These new approaches are sometimes known as standpoint perspectives because they express a view from the standpoint of a specifically defined social group.

A key argument of the standpoint perspectives is that the more established 'structure' and 'action' approaches within sociology have not recognised the significance of cultural diversity and social change within British society. Such mainstream sociological approaches are criticised for generating undifferentiated and culturally biased sociological analyses and findings and for applying them inappropriately to all social groups. In contrast, standpoint perspectives contribute the 'voices' and perspectives of less powerful social and cultural groups who feel that their experiences are marginalised and not recognised or represented within mainstream sociology. An awareness of standpoint perspectives is important and useful when thinking sociologically about health-care issues because they direct us to new issues and topics that are significant for many service users.

Feminist perspectives

A variety of different **feminist** perspectives have been developed to analyse and account for women's health experiences. Marxist feminists use the basic conflict model of Marxism to explain how women are exploited both in terms of social class and as women in a male-dominated society. This feminist perspective offers a structural, conflict viewpoint of society. Radical feminists view society primarily in terms of the conflict of interests and fundamental differences in power between men and women in society. The main argument of this approach is that society is patriarchal and works to ensure that male dominance is perpetuated at the expense of women. Finally, liberal feminists are concerned with achieving equality of opportunity in the society that we have rather than in overturning the current social system. They identify sexual discrimination as a major barrier to women's equality and try to change social processes and relationships to counteract this.

Anti-racist perspectives

Anti-**racist** perspectives understand and explain society from the perspective of minority ethnic groups. The key argument is that society is racially structured and works to protect the interests of the dominant white majority at the cost of minority ethnic groups. As such, anti-racist perspectives see racial discrimination at individual, institutional and societal levels as playing a powerful role in determining the life chances and experiences of non-white individuals and social groups. The policy goal of anti-racist sociologists is to challenge and change social processes and relationships that are based on racial discrimination.

⚷ *Keywords*

Feminism

This term generally refers to sociological and philosophical perspectives that examine the social world from the viewpoint of women.

⚷ *Keywords*

Racism

Ideas and beliefs about 'race' that are applied in a negative way, through unfair and less favourable treatment and hostility towards members of supposed 'racial groups'. The term is synonymous with 'racial discrimination'.

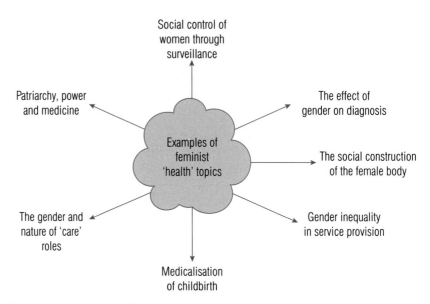

Figure 3.2 *Examples of feminist health topics*

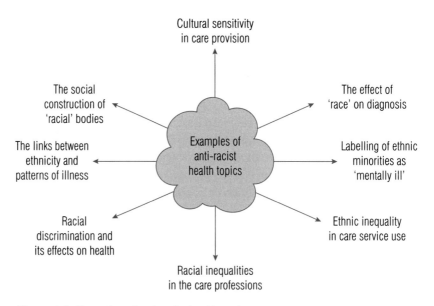

Figure 3.3 *Examples of anti-racist health topics*

Reflective activity

Reflect on the health-care setting where you work or where you have recently had a learning placement. Are there any aspects of your work, the care setting or patient experiences within it that could be analysed and understood using naturalistic, micro-sociological approaches?

Rapid recap

Check your progress so far by working through each of the following questions.

1. Identify two ways of approaching health-care issues sociologically.
2. Explain the difference between a social structure and a social action focus within sociology.
3. Describe the main concerns of feminist and anti-racist standpoint perspectives within sociology.

If you have difficulty with more than one of the questions, read through the section again to refresh your understanding before moving on.

References

Daykin, N. (2001) Sociological approaches to health, in *Health Care Studies* (eds. J. Naidoo and J. Wills). Palgrave Macmillan, Basingstoke.

Further reading

Haralambos, M. and Holborn, M. (2004) *Sociology – Themes and Perspectives*, 6th edn. Collins Education, London.

Seidman, S. (2004) *Contested Knowledge – Social Theory Today*, 3rd edn. Blackwell Publishing, Oxford.

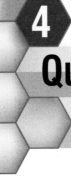

4

Questioning medical knowledge

Learning outcomes

By the end of this chapter you should be able to:

- Identify and describe the origins, development and main principles of the biomedical approach to health and illness

- Explain how sociological thinking can be used to challenge the biomedical approach to health and illness

- Understand sociological approaches that identify 'health' and 'illness' as social constructs.

Taking on the biomedical model

Sociological thinking has played a significant part in the questioning of medical knowledge. In some respects, the sociology of health and illness is a sceptical response to, and critique of, what is commonly known as the medical model of health and illness (see Nettleton 1998 and Higgs 2003 for further discussion of this point). A more current term for the medical model is the *biomedical* model of health and illness. The latter term draws our attention more clearly to the biological basis and 'logic' of this approach to health and illness.

The biomedical model is now the dominant theoretical approach to health and illness in Western societies (and the developed world). It claims to offer superior, or inherently more correct, ways of understanding health and illness issues compared to other approaches. Its claims to supremacy are founded on its scientific credentials and its 'objective' methods of diagnosing and treating a wide range of health problems.

However, in order to think sociologically about biomedical science we need to understand its emergence and dominance culturally and historically. This will enable us to appreciate its contemporary significance in the health field more fully. We will also consider how and why sociological critics of the medical profession question the claims and credibility of biomedicine as a way of diagnosing and curing health problems and argue that they are overstated and, in reality, limited.

Medicine and medical practice in health care

The biomedical model informs the approach to health knowledge and health-care practice of most medical practitioners, many paramedical professionals and a significant proportion of the general public in Britain. Because the biomedical model is so powerful and dominant in Western health-care systems, it can be difficult to believe that it is a relatively recent way of thinking about and practising health care, or that a range of credible alternatives to it exist.

The emergence of the medical profession

Ideas about health and health-care practices have a very long history. The ways in which people have thought about health, and have used these ideas to try to influence life-cycle and disease processes, is sometimes presented as a linear process of ongoing improvement and progress from simple, unsophisticated beginnings until complex, scientific medicine as we know it today emerged. While modern medicine does draw on earlier ideas about health, it is important to clarify what its scientific approach involves and to locate its emergence in a broader social and historical context.

A number of significant changes took place in the social, political and intellectual fields during the 18th and 19th centuries. These established the social, political and intellectual conditions in which medicine as a system of thought and a health-care practice was able to emerge. As well as changes in the way in which people lived and worked, there was a significant shift in the way in which people thought about issues such as health. Religion provided the dominant system of knowledge, or way of thinking about and explaining phenomena such as health and illness, in the pre-Enlightenment 17th century. People explained and understood the world, and their existence within it, in terms of 'the will of God' and divine intervention. Scientific thought emerged out of the Enlightenment, and gradually became the dominant system of knowledge during the 18th and 19th centuries.

Science, developed by people such as doctors, became the new source of 'truth', taking over from God. In the 18th and 19th centuries, medicine was a new scientific way of thinking about and dealing with health matters. Doctors claimed that they could use the scientific method objectively to identify and deal with ill health. They did this by developing techniques and procedures that applied positivist, scientific thinking to the care of the sick individual's body.

Science became the dominant system of knowledge during the 19th century, and remained a very powerful and important way of thinking about the world throughout the 20th century. This has enabled doctors to establish and maintain control over the way in

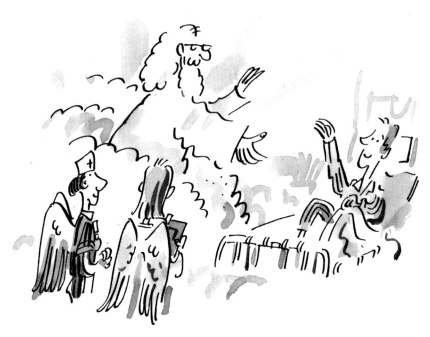

The god-like power of some doctors has a social history that can be traced back to the 18th century when science took over from religion as the source of truth about 'health' and health care

which health and illness are defined, and has strongly influenced the development of our present health-care system.

Medicine and 'disease'

Disease is a key concept in medicine. The ability to diagnose and treat disease is a central claim of medical practitioners. The biomedical approach to disease has its roots in molecular biology. It is mainly concerned with objectively identifying the organic (anatomical, physiological, biochemical) deviations that a disease presents from a measurable biological 'norm'. The biomedical methods of doctors are **objective** in the sense that they claim to provide ways of directly observing and measuring the signs of disease using scientific knowledge and techniques. Biopsies, physiological tests and physical examinations are all ways of putting this principle into practice. Medical practitioners claim that their knowledge of medicine gives them a superior way of diagnosing and treating the many forms of disease that they believe are the root of human health problems. As a result the medical profession, using a biomedical model of health that is actually founded on the concept of disease, has grown to dominate Western health-care practices and ways of thinking about health and illness.

⚬━ᴛ Keywords

Objective
Used to refer either to something that is unbiased (an objective opinion) or to something that exists in the real world outside the human mind. The biomedical approach to 'disease' makes use of both these meanings of the term.

Assumptions of the biomedical model of health

- The human body is a 'fixable machine'
- 'Health' is lost or affected when the body malfunctions, is damaged or functions abnormally
- The causes of health problems are located within the individual human body at a biological level
- The biomedical model refers to pathological (abnormal changes) in the body's structure or functioning as 'disease'
- Each 'disease' is seen as having specific biological causes – the doctrine of specific aetiology
- Western medical practitioners claim that disease processes can be diagnosed objectively by the use of scientific (anatomical, biochemical) methods
- Only medically trained professionals have the expertise to identify and diagnose health problems.

Over to you

Identify as many physical indicators of 'health' that you believe can be observed objectively using medical or other scientific techniques.

As well as claiming that 'disease' has an objective, biologically based impact on human health, the biomedical model also proposes that disease processes often occur naturally and independently of social behaviour or social influences. Consequently, people who show the signs or symptoms of a disease may be seen as being unlucky or as the unwitting victims of a genetically inherited 'time bomb' or *fait accompli* that they could have done little, and perhaps nothing, to avoid or change. In this way, biomedicine individualises both the causes and the experience of health problems in the concept and aetiology of 'disease'. However, sociological thinkers who are sceptical of individualised explanations (see Chapter 2, p. 14) that neglect social context and broader patterns of experience are likely to dispute this account of disease and medicine's claim to superior knowledge in the health field.

Medicine and 'illness'

What is the difference between 'illness' and 'disease'? Eisenberg (1977) distinguishes between them by saying that 'patients suffer "illnesses"; physicians diagnose and treat "disease" . . . illnesses are experienced as disvalued changes in states of being and social function: diseases are abnormalities in the structure and function of body organs and systems'. Helman (1981, p. 544) puts it clearly but slightly differently, saying that 'disease is something that an organ has: illness is something a man [sic] has'.

'Illness' is more problematic for the biomedical model than 'disease' because it refers to a **subjective** experience of 'ill health' or 'unwellness'. Sometimes this might be the consequence of having a 'disease'. At other times it can be a sense of lower or impaired functioning – feeling 'rough' or 'under the weather' to use common expressions. Illness is about how a person feels. As a result it is (culturally) valued as less important or significant than 'disease'. This last point alludes to the social nature of illness. The meaning of 'illness' is determined by the cultural context in which it occurs. Definitions of illness rely on social definitions of 'normality' and are much more problematic for doctors to pronounce on or determine. Popular definitions of 'illness' sometimes coincide with medical definitions of biological 'normality' but sometimes they don't. The important point to note is that 'illnesses' are culturally specific. It is usually the individual's use of a culturally specific definition of 'illness', not their experience of 'disease', that leads them to decide whether or not to seek help – perhaps even consulting health workers.

Keywords

Subjective
Used to refer to thoughts and ideas that are based on personal feelings or beliefs rather than on evidence found in the 'real' world. It is usually contrasted with objective.

Over to you

Identify examples of occasions where you've felt 'ill' or 'unwell' but were not suffering, objectively, from a 'disease'. How do you explain the causes of these experiences? What were other people's reactions to your subjective self-diagnosis of 'illness'?

Challenges to the biomedical model

For sociologists the experience of sickness and disease is an outcome of the organisation of society.

White 2002, p. 1

The medical profession, and the biomedical model that it draws on, have experienced a lot of criticism and challenges since the mid-1960s. Many of the challenges have been based on sociological criticisms of the biomedical model itself. Others have criticised and challenged the way in which medical practitioners have sought to extend their influence and expertise into areas of social behaviour and experience that have no apparent biomedical links. The social and political critiques of biomedicine and the medical profession have challenged the nature, uses and effects of medical knowledge and power in contemporary society.

The social construction of medical knowledge

Sociological critics who argue that 'diseases' are not real or naturally occurring phenomena but are in fact the products of social reasoning and social practices fundamentally challenge the biomedical model of health. This kind of critique of the biomedical model of health is based on the notion that the ideas and 'realities' of biomedicine are really **social constructions** (see p. 26). This isn't the same thing as saying that biomedical knowledge is illusory or fundamentally untrue. Rather, it means that biomedicine should be seen as a form of belief system that makes sense of 'health' in a particular way within particular social, historical and cultural contexts. Initially the idea that 'diseases' are socially constructed, rather than biologically natural and stable entities, may be difficult to accept.

What sociological critics of the biomedical model are in fact saying is that the 'medical' mode of thought that people now use to make sense of certain physical experiences is socially and historically specific. Through medical translation these physical experiences become the signs and symptoms or evidence of specific 'diseases' or medical conditions. Sociological critics of biomedicine argue that there is a social process of 'disease' creation going on here. The same signs and symptoms won't necessarily have the same natural meaning outside Western social contexts where biomedicine is less dominant. It is also clear that medical ideas about 'disease' and the causes of health problems can and do vary and change over time and between cultures. In contrast to the claims of biomedicine, 'diseases' are therefore not always stable, biologically based realities. There are many examples of new diseases being identified as well as examples of diseases that have apparently disappeared over time in Western cultures. How can we explain this? Is it possible that the medical profession make regular 'scientific' discoveries that reveal new forms of 'disease' and also find ways of curing and eradicating other 'diseases'? Or is it possible that the medical profession is, in fact, socially constructing disease categories in response to social pressures and a concern to maintain its dominant power in the health field?

Recently discovered and vanished 'diseases'

Recently discovered 'diseases'

- 'Addictive personality'
- Attention deficit hyperactivity disorder (ADHD)
- Compulsive shopping disorder
- Munchausen's syndrome by proxy

'Diseases' that have disappeared

- Female hysteria
- Masturbatory insanity
- Homosexuality

Sociological critics of biomedicine have also noted that there are wholesale differences between the health belief models and treatment approaches of Western and non-Western societies. The reason for this is not that Western biomedicine is superior or that its non-Western counterparts offer inferior or simpler approaches to health and illness. The contrast arises, instead, from the social and cultural differences that are apparent in Western and non-Western societies. As a social construct, 'medical' knowledge reflects the patterns of thinking and the dominant sources of 'truth' in a society. In sociological terms, Western medical notions of 'disease' are, therefore, socially contingent not naturally occurring categories of knowledge.

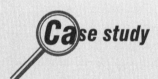

Case study

Robbins, J. M., Korda, H. and Shapiro, M. F. (1982) Treatment for a nondisease: the case of low blood pressure. *Social Science and Medicine*, **16**, 27–33.

This study documents diagnosis and treatment of hypotension in a sample of 1019 subjects. A quarter of this sample were diagnosed as hypotensive. Typically, these were older women with less education and low income. Although low blood pressure is harmless for the majority of people, 10% of the screened sample reported receiving treatment from their doctor for the condition. This typically consisted of harmless but ineffective placebo-like medicines including veal liver extract capsules or injections, iron capsules, tonics and vitamin B_{12}.

Medicine and social control

Since the 1970s the once-revered medical profession has been subject to increasing levels of criticism. While various parties, from governments to patients, have been involved in criticising the institution of medicine and medical practitioners themselves,

○━ᴛ *Keywords*

Patriarchy
A form of society in which men
have most of the power and
use it to rule and occupy
leadership positions.

sociological critics levelled some major social control accusations against biomedicine early on. In particular, sociological critics have questioned the idea that medicine is an area of health-care practice that is simply concerned with helping and caring for sick people. Instead, the institution of medicine has been criticised for being deeply **patriarchal** and for taking on a significant 'social control' role in contemporary society.

Elliot Freidson (1970) was one of the first sociological critics to question the social and political decision-making powers that medical practitioners often seemed to apply in their work with patients. Being able to officially define 'health' and 'sickness' in effect gave medical practitioners the right to define 'normality' and 'abnormality' in relation to a wide range of behaviours and experiences.

Medical practitioners have become very powerful by protecting their claim to 'superior' and privileged medical knowledge. According to their sociological critics this results in doctors frequently straying into areas of practice that have little to do with biomedicine and more to do with a desire for social and political power. The sociological critique suggests that in doing so doctors exercise moral judgements about particular groups of people, their lifestyles and forms of behaviour that offended social 'norms' rather than any kind of biomedical criteria. In this way the practice of medicine becomes a form of surveillance on society that is based on a spurious appeal to 'science'. For example, a number of 'disease' diagnoses appear to have more to do with judging and controlling people's behaviour than with any kind of biomedical reality. 'Masturbatory insanity' in the 17th century and women's 'hysteria' in the 19th century are historical examples. More contemporary examples could be said to include 'sex addiction', 'personality disorder', 'attention deficit hyperactivity disorder' (ADHD) and 'cannabis psychosis'.

The application of medical knowledge in relation to mental illness was, and still is, seen as a good example of the way that medical practitioners have used their privileged access to highly valued 'medical knowledge' for sociopolitical purposes. Critics, including mental health service users and 'survivors', argue that 'mental illness' diagnoses that are applied by medical practitioners have more of a social control purpose than any kind of 'health' function or 'scientific' validity (see Chapter 10 for more on this issue). In this sense, biomedical definitions of 'disease' and other ill health 'realities' are allegedly based as much on moral criteria and ethical judgements about 'normality' as on 'scientific' facts.

Medicalisation

Medicalisation is the term used within sociology to describe the process through which areas of social life have come under the medical gaze and have been 'colonised' by the medical profession.

Sociological critics of biomedicine use the concept of medicalisation to object to, and challenge, the expansion of medicine's social field of interest and power base. They argue that, throughout the 20th and into the 21st century, the medical profession has sought to apply medical knowledge to a range of non-biological areas of social life and experience. Areas such as ageing, childbirth, children's behaviour and substance misuse have all become the focus of medical 'expertise' and have been redefined as medical 'problems'. The recent 'discovery' of ADHD as a medical disorder provides a good example of medicalisation. Some present-day medical practitioners believe that ADHD results from a biochemical disorder within the child while others point to the way in which medical diagnosis judges a child's behaviour according to social criteria of what is acceptable and 'normal'.

White (2002) argues that through the medicalisation process doctors use the superior power of biomedicine to construct new medical realities out of previously non-medical situations. For example, childbirth has largely become a clinical safety issue since being medicalised whereas it was, for much longer in human history, a natural process controlled by women. Feminist critics of the medicalisation of childbirth argue that the real purpose and effect of medical dominance in the area of childbirth is to define and control women's roles and social experiences.

Questioning the effectiveness of medicine

One of the main themes in the conventional history of modern medicine is that it has developed into a highly effective way of dealing with health problems and has improved the quality of life and the longevity of the population in modern society. Sociological critics of biomedicine dispute this, arguing that medicine's efficacy has been overplayed. For example, McKeown (1976) is often quoted by sociological critics to demonstrate how the decline in mortality from infectious diseases since the 19th century has resulted more from social changes and public health initiatives than from developments in medical knowledge or practice.

Figure 4.1 clearly shows that death rates from respiratory tuberculosis had declined significantly, well before any medical discoveries were made to assist in its control. Tackling poor housing and providing clean water and sanitation systems appear to have

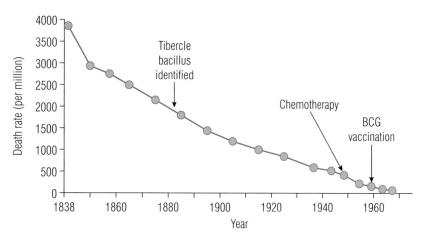

Figure 4.1 *Respiratory tuberculosis – death rates per million, England and Wales (from The Role of Medicine: Dream, Mirage or Nemesis?)*

been more important in reducing the mortality rates than developing effective chemotherapy for tuberculosis.

Ivan Illich (1976), a prominent American critic of the biomedical model, has also questioned the effectiveness of medicine on the grounds that medical practices actually cause harm. He refers to the harmful effects of medicine as their iatrogenic consequences. Illich (1976) is critical of medical practices for contributing to illness and damage to patients' health through, for example, the development and spread of methicillin-resistant *Staphylococcus aureus* (MRSA) infection in medical settings such as hospitals. Illich (1976) also argues that medicine has indirectly had a negative impact on health by deskilling people. That is, the 'expertise' of doctors and their close control of medical knowledge and treatment skills have undermined our general ability to manage our own health and well-being. We are now dependent on medical 'experts' to do so.

Arguably, the recent questioning of medical knowledge and the effectiveness of medical practices have led to a reduction of faith and trust in biomedicine and the medical profession in Western societies. One consequence has been an increasing demand for non-medical, alternative or complementary forms of health care and greater patient control over health and care processes.

Reflective activity

Taking both sociological criticism and your own knowledge and experiences into account, reflect on the extent to which you trust the medical profession and believe in the effectiveness of biomedicine. Think through the evidence that you base your judgement on.

Is the criticism of biomedicine justified?

Sociological critics of biomedicine have tended to use forms of social constructionism to contest and critique medical knowledge and medical power in the health field. In doing so they have tended to reject the 'empirical' or evidence basis of medicine. In exchange they offer a constructive epistemology that doesn't accept the existence of fixed, external realities. This can be problematic for health carers and service users to grasp and accept, given their experience of apparently real physical and mental health problems.

One of the responses that biomedical supporters make to their sociological critics is that social constructionism fails to acknowledge the real effects that biological mechanisms have on human health and well-being. This failure could be seen as undermining, or at best neglecting, the validity of people's experiences of pain, suffering and distress. Additionally, the social constructionist approach is criticised for underplaying the real improvements and achievements of modern medicine in tackling a wide range of physical and mental health problems.

The contribution of the medical model

I have outlined a number of ways in which medical knowledge and power have been questioned. Clearly, there are grounds for doubting that medicine can deliver 'health' for all in a simple, curative way. Nevertheless, given the power and importance of medicine, it is worth making the point that medical knowledge and medical practitioners do have an important role to play in developing physical treatments for identifiable biological 'diseases' and disorders. Pharmaceuticals and surgical interventions are now very sophisticated, and can improve and prolong a person's life in a situation in which 100 years ago they would have died or suffered much more. Clearly, biomedicine does have a very important role to play in 'fighting disease' and 'saving lives' but there are plenty of arguments and sources of evidence to show that it is useful only for a proportion of the 'health' problems that people face, rather than for the entire range.

With our sociological interests in mind, it is important to restate the point that the UK's health-care system has been developed to accommodate and support the dominant knowledge system and practices of the 'curative' medical profession. However, despite the power of the biomedical model and the medical profession, there is a growing interest in other ways of thinking about and providing 'health' care. The growth of interest in complementary therapies and public health has led, for example, to a shift towards social theories of 'health' and 'illness', and complementary therapy approaches to the provision of treatments.

Alternative approaches to the medical model

The biomedical model and the current hospital-based medical system are not the only ways of thinking about health and of providing health care. Other alternatives include public health medicine at one extreme and complementary therapies at the other. Both have recently begun to make a comeback in debates about health and how health care can be provided.

Public health medicine and the environment

During the 19th century, the tradition of public health medicine developed alongside, but separate from, the individualised, biological focus of the biomedical model tradition. Both shared a negative definition of health as being the absence of illness. However, the public health model attempted, through preventive methods such as improving water supplies and developing public housing programmes and health education campaigns, to prevent general ill health from occurring in society in the first place. The public health approach adopts a social model of health. The real causes and origins of ill health are seen as being located in the social and physical environment rather than in the individual. For example, poor housing and poverty are environmental factors that contribute to respiratory problems. The public health solution is better housing and programmes to tackle inequality and poverty. The biomedical solution consists of antibiotics to treat the pathology, or malfunctioning, occurring in the individual's respiratory system.

The public health tradition was very important in reducing ill health and premature death rates at the turn of the 20th century. McKeown (1976), as we've seen, has presented evidence to show that many infectious diseases declined as a result of public health interventions rather than new 'scientific' techniques of individual medical practitioners (see Figure 4.1). The social model of health continues to inform the efforts of public health reformers in the 21st century, who see social inequalities and environmental issues as central to effective health-care provision.

Complementary health and therapy models

Alternative, or complementary, therapies involve ways of thinking about the nature of health and ill health that are significantly different from the biomedical model approach. Complementary therapies include practices such as homeopathy, which uses a range of herbal remedies in different strengths to stimulate the body's own defences, and acupuncture, which involves the insertion of needles at stimulus points in the body to effect 'cures'. Both these and most other forms of complementary practices have no 'scientific' basis – indeed, they may actually fly in the face of 'rational' thinking. An example of this is reflexology. This therapy is based on the belief that by treating the foot all parts of the body can be healed. There is no biomedical evidence to suggest that this is possible, yet people claim that it works – as they do for the entire range of practices classified as 'complementary therapy'.

Practitioners of complementary therapies pursue a range of different beliefs about how their techniques work (Table 4.1) but generally they agree that the division of the body into a separate mind and a mechanical body – the basis of the biomedical model – is false. In complementary medicine, a remedy needs to involve both body and mind if it is to be effective.

The growth of complementary medicine has been so rapid that it is estimated that there are now over 100,000 therapists in the UK and that over 10% of the British population now use them.

Table 4.1 Complementary therapy ideas about 'health'	
Type of treatment	**Fundamental ideas**
Acupuncture	A form of alternative therapy that has its origins in ancient China. It involves needles being inserted into the body to restore the 'energy flow' necessary for *ying* and *yang* elements of *chi* to be in balance
Herbal medicine	Uses various herbs to provoke the body's natural protective responses as a treatment for various illnesses
Homeopathy	This is based on the principle that 'like is cured by like' and involves the patient being given a very small dose of a remedy that is vigorously shaken to improve its potency. The idea is that this then allows the body to build up a natural immunity to the substance (and cures the problem)
Reflexology	This therapy is based on the belief that different parts of the feet correspond to different organs and parts of the body. By applying pressure to the different parts of the feet, the body can be treated for various problems
Hypnotherapy	Patients are put in a trance-like state in which they are felt to be more receptive to suggestions about behaviour change (stopping smoking or overeating for example) or are more able to express repressed feelings. The idea is that they may retain these suggestions or benefit from the emotional release after the hypnosis is ended

Until recently, the medical profession had been hostile to complementary therapies, but the British Medical Association (a very powerful pressure group that represents the medical profession) has begun to accept that they can be part of a range of possible ways of combating ill health. Indeed, just under 50% of GPs are now providing, either directly or indirectly, complementary therapies, and 70% of health authorities are also purchasing complementary therapy services.

Reflective activity

Reflect on what you've learnt about sociological criticisms of medical knowledge and the medical profession. To what extent do they unsettle your existing beliefs about, and trust in, the biomedical approach to health care? How could you adapt your approach to health-care practice to take these criticisms into account?

Rapid recap

Check your progress so far by working through each of the following questions.

1. Identify when, and describe why, the biomedical model of health care emerged.
2. Outline three ways in which sociological critics have challenged the biomedical model of the medical profession.
3. Identify and describe two alternative approaches to the biomedical model of health care.

If you have difficulty with more than one of the questions, read through the section again to refresh your understanding before moving on.

References

Eisenberg, L. (1977) Disease and Illness: distinctions between professional and popular ideas of sickness. *Culture, Medicine and Psychiatry*, **1**, 9–23.

Freidson, E. (1970) *Profession of Medicine: A Study of the Sociology of Applied Knowledge*. Harper & Row, New York.

Helman, C. (1981) Disease versus illness in general practice. *Journal of the Royal College of General Practitioners*, **31**, 548–552.

Higgs, P. (2003) The limits and boundaries of medical knowledge, in *Sociology as Applied to Medicine* (ed. G. Scambler). W.B. Saunders, London.

Illich, I. (1976) *Limits to Medicine*. Marion Boyars, London.

McKeown, T. (1976) *The Role of Medicine: Dream, Mirage or Nemesis?* London Provincial Hospitals Trust, London.

Nettleton, S. (1998) *The Sociology of Health and Illness*. Polity Press, Cambridge.

White, K. (2002) *Sociology of Health and Illness*. Sage, London.

Further reading

Clarke, A. (2001) *The Sociology of Healthcare*. Prentice Hall, Harlow.

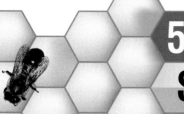

5

Social class and health experience

Learning outcomes

By the end of this chapter you should be able to:

- Describe the main sociological approaches to identifying and understanding social class in Britain
- Outline the main patterns of health and illness experience according to social class in Britain
- Discuss possible explanations for the link between social class and health experience.

🔑 *Keywords*

Longitudinal

A type of research design in which a sample of people provide data on a number of separate occasions over a relatively long period of time.

Social class

A term used to identify a group of people who are similar in terms of their wealth, income and occupation. Social classes are seen to exist in a hierarchical structure.

Social class and health experience

What is 'social class'? How is a person's social class linked to their health experience? These are the two main questions that we'll be addressing in this chapter. The possible links between social class and health have been an area of controversy and considerable interest to both the health-care and the sociological community for many years. In particular, the possibility that illness patterns and death rates are affected by the social class structure of British society is a major issue for service planners and health-care practitioners as well as those sections of the population who experience most social disadvantage.

The social structure of British society

Social structure is a key concept within sociology. Sociological approaches to the human world that focus on social structures are, not surprisingly, called 'structuralist' approaches. These approaches see 'social structure' as 'networks of social institutions and social relationships which are comparatively lasting and which do not change with the coming and going of the particular individuals who form them' (Taylor and Field 1997, p. 17). In the health field, structural approaches tend to consider how the structuring of society influences patterns of health and illness experience and the collective, organised response to it. As a result sociological research into these issues tends to be based on large-scale, often **longitudinal**, surveys and analyses of mortality (death) and morbidity (illness) rates and patterns.

Health-care practitioners who are interested in the relationships between social structure and patterns of health and illness experience can conceptualise 'social structure' in a number of different ways. Perhaps the most well-known way is to think of 'society' as being organised and structured around **social classes**. Britain has long been seen as a class-based society, although the importance and impact of social class on a person's life chances generally, and their health experiences specifically, is also the subject of a lot of dispute.

For many sociologists the existence of a social class hierarchy in British society has the most profound effect on a person's life chances and is the main way in which society is socially stratified and divided. Sociologists interested in the health field have certainly made social class a priority when investigating the relationships between social structure and patterns of health and illness (see p. 56). However, British society can also be seen as being structured and organised around a range of other social divisions. For example, the sociological and specialist health literature also identifies age structures, gender structures (see p. 70) and ethnicity structures (see p. 86), as elements in the social stratification of society.

Over to you

Are you conscious of your 'social class' background or the 'social class' status of your family? How would you describe this and how does (or why doesn't) it affect your life?

Why does social stratification matter?

The point of identifying the ways in which society is stratified and divided goes beyond the goal of making an adequate description of social structure. Often those who focus on the relationships between social structure and health also have a political motivation to reveal the impact that social inequality has on different social groups. In the health field, for example, social researchers and health-care practitioners have sought to draw attention to the ways in which health and illness experiences follow social class, gender and ethnicity patterns. Establishing that health and illness experiences are socially patterned then opens up a whole range of new questions about why this is so and what can, and should be, done about it.

Theory into Practice

Government health-care policy often accepts, and is a response to, the notion that social inequality exists in British society. One common policy strategy is to target resources and services at those groups who are seen as the most socially disadvantaged and therefore 'in need'.

There is a continuing debate within the sociology community, as well as in health-care and political circles, about the extent to which social structure affects 'life chances'. At one extreme, people argue that various aspects of social structure are so powerful that they largely determine the opportunities and life experiences that we are likely to have. The alternative position criticises this 'iron cage' image of social structure and argues that we can escape from, or act outside of, the effects of social structure to shape our own destiny in contemporary society. The dispute between these two positions is known as the 'structure/agency' debate. It lies at the heart of sociology's fundamental interest in the relationship between the individual and society.

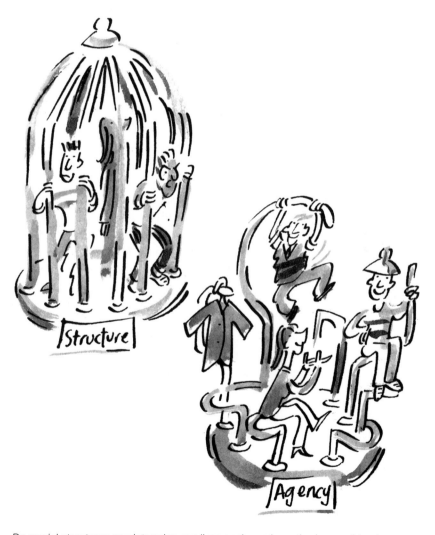

Do social structures predetermine our lives or do we have the 'agency' to shape our own destiny?

> *Over to you*
>
> What contribution do you think health-care workers can make if social structure really is largely responsible for determining an individual's life chances?

The emergence of social class

The concept of social class is used to identify groups of people who are similar in terms of their wealth, income and occupations. Sociologists argue that the current social class system emerged as a result of the development of capitalism and the decline of the feudal ordering of British society from the early 19th century onwards.

Britain's feudal society was rigidly stratified. A person's position in the feudal system depended on their ownership, or non-ownership, of land and their relationship to the monarch (king or queen). The monarch was at the very top of the social hierarchy and owned all of the land in Britain. The king had the right to distribute land to members of the aristocracy, who lay beneath him in the feudal hierarchy. Land was then leased or rented to people further down the hierarchy. However, there was always a significantly large group of ordinary people, the peasants or serfs, who had little economic power because they owned no land in what was an agricultural economy. Ordinary people owed their loyalty and allegiance to their land-owning 'superiors' and had little or no opportunity to acquire land or improve their social position. As a result very little social mobility occurred in Britain's feudal society until the emergence of a capitalist economic system.

The capitalist economic system emerged during Britain's industrial revolution in the late 18th and 19th centuries. It transformed feudalistic social relations in Britain. This was because industrial employers were able to develop new employment relationships with workers that didn't involve any kind of 'feudal' duty to a powerful landowner. However, a new 'social class' hierarchy did emerge out of this capitalist economic system. This was based on a person's occupation and the social status or prestige that this had in society. People who had highly sought-after and prestigious occupations belonged to higher social classes and people whose occupations were not prestigious belonged to lower classes. A further consequence of the new economic basis of social relations was that upward social mobility became possible because people were able to work their way up (or slip down!) the social class structure. Social position was no longer determined by birth.

Ways of thinking about 'social class'

The above account of the way that social classes emerged in Britain is inevitably simplified. However, you should note that a person's occupation, or socioeconomic position, is generally seen by sociologists as being the key variable (but not the only factor) that 'positions' them within a hierarchical social class, or socioeconomic, structure. Even so, there are a number of different ways of conceptualising, or thinking about, the nature of the social class structure in British society today.

The three-class pyramid

The classic way of thinking about social class in Britain is to identify the working class, the middle class and the upper class as the three distinct social classes. In this model, the working class forms the largest social group at the base of the social class hierarchy or pyramid (Figure 5.1). The main characteristic of people in this social class is that they, or the head of their household, have a manual occupation. By contrast the smaller proportion of people who make up the middle class are identified as people who belong to a household where the (usually male) head has a non-manual occupation. The upper class is a relatively small proportion of people who are wealthy, powerful and have a lot of social status.

This three-tier social class pyramid provides a relatively crude way of looking at the way in which social stratification occurs on economic grounds. While it is acknowledged that each social class has 'within-class' economic differences, other methods of classifying people into social classes are based on more wide-ranging and subtle criteria.

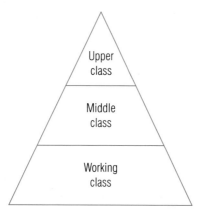

Figure 5.1 *The three-class pyramid*

The Registrar General's scale

The social classification system used until 2001 to identify and record an individual's social class was known as the Registrar General's scale. Statistics based on this scale were developed from national census records, which provided details of the occupation of the head of each household in Britain. The scale consisted of six social classes (Table 5.1), which were organised into a hierarchy that linked occupation to social status. This hierarchy was, once again, perceived in terms of a social class pyramid (Figure 5.2).

At the beginning of the 21st century, the Registrar General's scale was felt to be out of date and an inadequate method of classifying the class structure of modern Britain. A new scale was developed for use in the 2001 census.

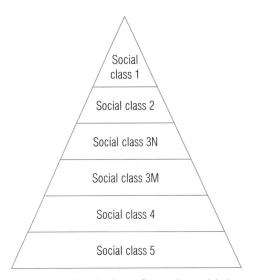

Figure 5.2 *The Registrar General's social class pyramid*

Table 5.1 The Registrar General's social class scale	
Social class	**Types of occupation**
Class 1 – Professional occupations	Lawyers, doctors
Class 2 – Intermediate occupations	Social workers, managers, shopkeepers
Class 3N – Skilled, non-manual occupations	Clerks, policemen, nurses
Class 3M – Skilled, manual occupations	Electricians, coal miners
Class 4 – Partly skilled occupations	Nursing assistants, farm workers, bus drivers
Class 5 – Unskilled	Porters, cleaners

The National Statistics socioeconomic classification

The National Statistics socioeconomic classification (NS-SEC) system has been developed to incorporate the changes that occurred in Britain's class structure over the last few decades of the 20th century. The main change involved expanding the classification system to reflect the growth of middle-class occupations and the changing nature of the kinds of work that people do as well as the levels of social esteem that these jobs attract. This results in more of a diamond-shaped image of the social class structure (Figure 5.3). There are now eight major social classes in the NS-SEC scale (Table 5.2).

Does social class still matter?

Sociologists recognise that social class is not as important in the way that people define themselves or construct their social identities as it used to be. The fact that society appears to be becoming more socially and ethnically differentiated suggests that there are fewer major distinctions within the population (such as between working and middle class people) than was previously the case. However, despite the suggestions of some politicians, Britain is far from being a 'classless society'. Social class may play less of a role in our sense of personal identity and we may be less aware of status distinctions in contemporary society. However, this does not mean that the structural effects of social class have necessarily diminished. Data

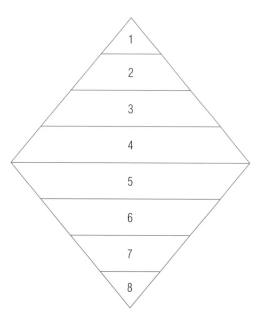

Figure 5.3 *The National Statistics socioeconomic classification diamond structure*

Table 5.2 NS-SEC social class classification system

Social class	Types of jobs included
1. Higher managerial and professional occupations	Doctors, lawyers, dentists, professors, professional engineers
2. Lower managerial and professional occupations	School teachers, nurses, journalists, actors, police sergeants
3. Intermediate occupations	Airline cabin crew, secretaries, photographers, fire fighters, auxiliary nurses
4. Small employers and own account workers	Self-employed builders, hairdressers fishermen, car dealers and shop owners
5. Lower supervisory and technical occupations	Train drivers, employed craftsmen, foremen, supervisors
6. Semi-routine occupations	Shop assistants, postal workers, security guards
7. Routine occupations	Bus drivers, waiters and waitresses, cleaners, car park attendants, refuse collectors
8. Never worked or long-term unemployed	Students, people not classifiable, occupations not stated

from the national census and other research investigations shows that there is a socioeconomic hierarchy in Britain and that this affects 'life chances' in various ways.

Many sociologists and health-care practitioners believe that social class is the key form of social stratification in modern society. Sociological research has repeatedly shown that social class has a greater effect on a person's life chances than other important social variables such as gender, ethnicity, age or experience of disability. This doesn't mean that these other features of social stratification are not important in modern British society. However, their impact should always be considered alongside an individual's social class position.

Social class and health experience

Why do health-care workers always ask patients about their occupation when they're assessing their physical or mental health problems? Does it help to know that the person is a builder or a lawyer? What do we gain from obtaining this kind of information? Arguably, there are a variety of reasons for finding out what kind of work (paid and unpaid) a person does. For example, knowledge of a person's occupation may reveal something about the risks associated with their work and might also provide some insight into their (probable) lifestyle and their material circumstances. These latter insights would be based, to a large degree, on supposition and assumptions about different occupations and the social groups that typically perform them. However, it is also the case that, if we are able to identify a person's occupation, we may be able to make use of sociological research on the links between occupationally defined social class and consistent patterns of health and illness experience.

Remember that sociologists tend to argue that a person's experience of health and illness is not simply the result of biological factors or 'chance'. From a sociological perspective, health and illness are 'social', not individual, matters. In particular, researchers using sociological methods have presented a wide range of data to show that significant and enduring patterns of health and illness experience are linked to social class.

Social class patterns of mortality

Sociologists have conducted a large number of research studies on the possible effects of social class on life chances. A persistent finding is that a person's social class is the most important predictor of health experience and mortality (death). The key finding that is regularly revealed by sociological data from these studies is that there is a social class gradient in mortality. There is a steplike pattern of increasing mortality from the highest down to the lowest social class. The **mortality rate** of the lowest social class is approximately twice that of the highest social class. In essence, people in the higher social classes live longer than people in the lower social classes.

Richard Wilkinson, a sociological researcher, wrote a letter in 1976 to a social science journal called *New Society* about this apparent connection. He asked the Labour government of the time to set up an urgent inquiry into the causes of the link between social class, health experience and death rates. The Black Report of 1980 (Townsend *et al.* 1988) was the result of the inquiry. This produced hard, empirical evidence of considerable social class differences in health experiences.

The Black Report also showed that differences in death rates between those at the top, and those at the bottom, of the social class hierarchy had increased during the 20th century despite the emergence of the National Health Service in the 1940s. For example, in 1930 unskilled workers were 23% more likely to die prematurely than professional workers. By 1970, the likelihood had increased to 61%. The report was very controversial and was initially

⊙━┳ *Keywords*

Mortality rate
The number of people dying, within a particular period, per 100,000 of the population.

Standardised mortality rate (SMR)
A mortality rate that assumes the average risk of death for all 16–65-year-olds in the population to be 100. Social groups with an SMR score above 100 have a higher risk of early death within a specified period and social groups with an SMR below 100 have a lower risk.

Table 5.3 Social class and mortality rates in England and Wales, 1991–95 (data from Drever and Whitehead 1997)

Social class	Stillbirth rate	Infant mortality rate	Mortality rate 1–15 years	SMR (men, 20–64 years)
1	4	4	18	66
2	4	5	16	72
3N	5	5	16	100
3M	5	6	26	117
IV	6	7	22	116
V	8	8	42	189

suppressed by Conservative governments in the 1980s. However, to some sociologists and policy makers this kind of finding provides powerful and compelling evidence of the influence and impact of large-scale structural forces on health and illness experience in British society.

Debates about the social class patterning of health and illness experience have centred on, and often refer back to, the findings of the pioneering Black Report. The report remains significant because it was the first sociological study to provide detailed empirical data showing a social class gradient in health and illness experience. It showed that the lower a person's social class the more likely they were to experience ill health and to die at an early age. The report showed that in 1980 unskilled workers were still two and a half times more likely to die before retirement than professional workers. More recent data show that, over the past 20 years, death rates have fallen across all social groups and for both sexes. Despite this, the chances of people from the higher social classes dying early are still falling faster than those of people from lower social classes.

In the early 1970s, the mortality rate among males of working age was twice as high in the lowest social class as in the highest. By the late 1990s, the figure was *three* times higher! Life expectancy at birth for men belonging to social classes I and II (Registrar General's scale) increased by 2 years during the 1980s, yet for classes IV and V the increase was only 1.4 years. Men could expect to live to 75 in the higher social classes but only to 70 in the lower classes. Women could expect to live to 80 in the higher social classes but only to 77 in the lower classes. At present, 5 out of every 1000 infants from parents in the two higher social classes die at birth but 7 out of every 1000 infants from parents in the two lower social classes die at birth. Statistics like these consistently show that mortality rates are socially patterned.

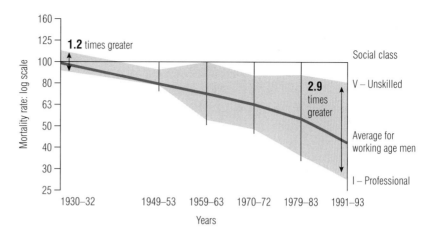

Figure 5.4 *The widening mortality gap between the classes (redrawn from Office for National Statistics 2001)*

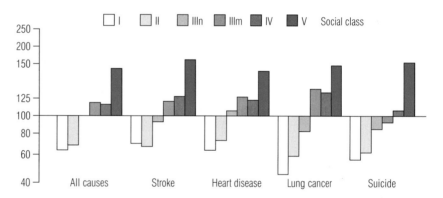

Figure 5.5 *Social class and major causes of death (redrawn from* Social Sciences *29 June 1997 Her Majesty's Stationery Office)*

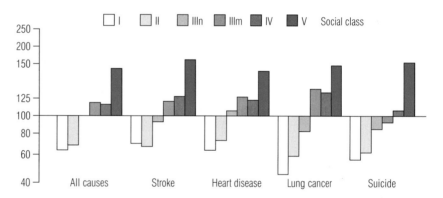

Figure 5.5 *Social class and major causes of death (redrawn from* Social Sciences *29 June 1997 Her Majesty's Stationery Office)*

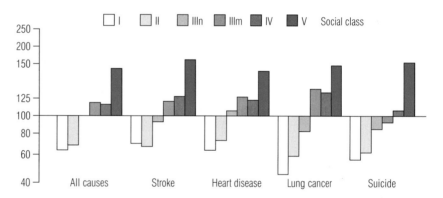 Keywords

Morbidity rates
Reported patterns of illness and disease. Sources can include self-reported illness experience as well as statistics compiled from hospital visits and GP appointments.

Social class patterns of morbidity

Unlike mortality rates, **morbidity rates** have not declined over the last 20 years. The most recent figures show that 17% of professional men aged 45–64 years of age reported a 'limited long-standing illness' (chronic illness), compared to a much larger 48% of unskilled males. For women of the same age, 25% of professional, and 45% of unskilled, women workers disclosed chronic illness. Obesity is a commonly used measure of poor health, as it is linked to heart problems. A total of 25% of women and 18% of men in class V were obese compared to 14% of women and 11% of men in social class I. Women in lower social classes are also more likely to experience mental illness than women in higher social classes.

> ## Over to you
>
> * Do you think that health-care workers should take social class into account in their assessment of an individual's health problems and future health needs?
> * How do you think this could be done in your work place or intended area of practice?

Explaining the links between social and health experience

Sociologists, and many health-care workers, view studies that identify links between social class and health experience as a significant achievement in the use and application of sociological methods. However, we need to be careful about what the data actually tells us. Many of the sociological studies that provide evidence of a link between social class and health leave open the issue of why this link exists. All they reveal is that there does appear to be a link. But what causes it? There are a number of different, and partly competing, explanations. The Black Report outlined four different ways of explaining the relationship between health and social status:

* **The artefact approach** claims that the apparent gap between the higher and lower social classes is a result only of the way that data is sought and collected and is not a 'true' picture. The results are therefore an 'artefact', or effect, of sociologists' data collection methods, not of any link between class and health!
* **The social selection explanation** is that those people who are 'fitter' and in better health are more able to obtain better jobs, and *vice versa*. The statistics do show that people in poor health are more likely to be unemployed or in lower-paid occupations. Downward social mobility is partly related to chronic ill health.
* **Cultural explanations** stress that lifestyle choices (about exercise, diet, smoking and alcohol use, for example) made by individuals and different social groups affect their subsequent health and illness experience.
* **Structural explanations** argue that it is not personal choice but social structures that determine lifestyle and establish the key links to health experience. For example, people who experience low income or poverty, work and relationship pressures, poor housing and oppressive work conditions are seen as the victims of structural inequalities in British society rather than as bad decision-makers.

The Acheson Report (1998), a relatively recent investigation into inequalities in health, was very sympathetic to the two final explanations suggested by the Black Report. However, Sir Donald Acheson's report provided a more subtle and sophisticated explanation for apparent inequalities in health experience. The Acheson Report saw it as the result of a complex interweaving between individual biological factors, individual personalities, lifestyle choices and the necessities imposed by income and employment. The key point that the report makes is that individual health is the result of a complex set of wider cultural and economic factors that interact with a series of personal choices based on biological and psychological influences.

Social capital and health experience

Explanation of the apparent social class gradient in morbidity and mortality remains unresolved. While many health-care practitioners and sociologists are prepared to accept the 'combination of factors' point made in the Acheson Report, their attention has turned more recently to the concept of social capital. But what is 'social capital'?

Putnam (1995) says:

'By social capital I mean features of social life – networks, norms, and trust – that enable participants to act together more effectively to pursue shared objectives . . . To the extent that the norms, networks and trust link substantial sectors of the community and span underlying cleavages . . . those who have wider and more closely integrated social networks . . . feel a sense of well-being.'

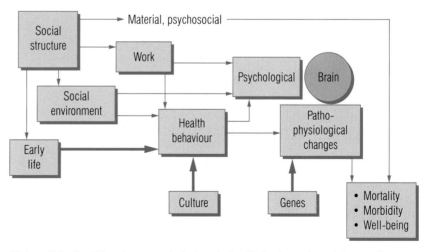

Figure 5.6 *Social and economic factors in health (redrawn from Acheson Report 1998)*

Richard Wilkinson (1996) draws on the concept of social capital when he argues that a high degree of income inequality in a rich country makes social divisions worse, reduces levels of trust and the quality of community life and increases social anxiety and stress levels. As a result the 'social environment' of the country becomes more hostile and less hospitable, leading to poorer health and greater social exclusion for those with least income and wealth. In this way, Wilkinson moves the analysis of health inequalities beyond a focus purely on social class without diminishing its importance as a feature of a culture of inequality to which poor health experience appears to be linked.

Reflective activity

Reflect on the insights that have been provided by sociological studies into the relationship between social class structures and health experience. How can you make use of these in your own health-care practice? Do the ways of explaining the links between social class and health help you to understanding service users' health and illness experiences?

Rapid recap

Check your progress so far by working through each of the following questions.

1. Define the terms morbidity, mortality and standardised mortality rate.
2. Describe three ways of conceptualising Britain's social class structure.
3. Outline the key finding of sociological studies into the link between social class and health experience and identify four explanations for it.

If you have difficulty with more than one of the questions, read through the section again to refresh your understanding before moving on.

References

Acheson Report (1998) Independent Inquiry into Inequalities in Health: Report. The Stationery Office, London.

Drever, F. and Whitehead, M. (1997) *Health inequalities*. Office for National Statistics, London.

Office for National Statistics (2001) Tackling health inequalities: a programme for action. Stationery Office, London.

Putnam, R. D. (1995) *Bowling Alone: The Collapse and Revival of American Community*. Simon & Schuster, New York.

Taylor, S. and Field, D. (1997) *Sociology of Health and Health Care*. Oxford, Blackwell.

Townsend, P., Davidson, N. and Whitehead, M. (eds.) (1988) *Inequalities in Health: The Black Report and the Health Divide*. Penguin, Harmondsworth.

Wilkinson, R. G. (1996) *Unhealthy Societies: The Afflictions of Inequality*. Routledge, London.

Further reading

Naidoo, J. and Wills, J. (2001) *Health Studies – An Introduction*. Palgrave, Basingstoke.

Nettleton, S. (1995) *The Sociology of Health and Illness*. Polity Press, Cambridge.

Walsh, M., Stephens, P. and Moore, S. (2000) *Social Policy and Welfare*. Nelson Thornes, Cheltenham.

Miers, M. (2003) *Class, Inequalities and Nursing Practice.* Palgrave Macmillan, Basingstoke.

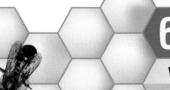

6

Women, gender and health

⚬━ᴛ *Keywords*

....

Gender
The cultural and social attributes or expectations of men and women in society that are expressed through notions of masculinity and femininity.

Women's health matters

One of the most significant areas of social change in the 20th century was the changing role of women in society. Sociologists, particularly those who developed and used feminist perspectives, played a significant part in supporting women's struggle for equality of opportunity and equal legal rights with men throughout the last century and continue to do so. Since the 1960s, significant feminist campaigns have focused on the status, rights and experiences of women across a broad range of areas of social life. Women's access to appropriate health-care services, their significant role in care provision and gender differences in patterns of mortality and morbidity have all attracted the attention of sociologists and health-care practitioners who are interested in the particular health experiences of women. In this chapter, we will focus on the sociological aspects of each of these issues and their implications for health-care practice.

The limitations of 'sex' (and importance of 'gender')

Sociologists make a distinction between the terms 'sex' and '**gender**'. 'Sex' tends to be used to refer to the specific, but limited, biological differences between men and women. 'Gender', by contrast, is used to identify and acknowledge ways in which men and women are differently constituted as social subjects by social and political forces in contemporary society. As such, we need to ensure that we locate our discussions, and subsequent understanding, of women's health issues, in the context of gender relations and women's ongoing struggle against gender inequality.

Contesting the 'natural' role of women

One of the main obstacles that women had to overcome in their campaign for equality of opportunity in education and work was the notion that a woman's 'natural' role is that of housewife, mother and 'carer'. For many decades this cultural expectation acted as a barrier to equality of opportunity for women. While the idea that men and women have different 'natural' roles in life because of their different biological characteristics hasn't entirely disappeared, it is less prevalent. The idea was, and still is, a reflection of certain attitudes, norms and values that exist in society generally. Women are seen as 'natural' carers in situations where their childbearing potential is used to define their 'essential' social role. What results is a **stereotype** – the housewife, mother and 'carer' – that fails to see broader social, political and economic possibilities for women or to question taken-for-granted gender relations that define women in a secondary, supportive role to a male 'breadwinner'.

Sociologists, particularly those using feminist perspectives, have long contested the 'natural carer' claim by using sociological concepts such as socialisation, gender and stereotyping to explain how individuals learn to behave and relate to others in 'gendered' ways. The significance of inborn biological differences between men and women has been so widely contested since the 1960s, when feminism became a powerful sociological perspective, that most people now accept that male and female members of society should enjoy equality of opportunity.

> ## Over to you
>
> - Identify the different ways in which you have experienced gender **socialisation**.
> - What attributes or behaviours do others expect of you because of your gender?
> - How do gender stereotypes inform the expectations that people have about different health-care roles?

Thinking about gender relations

So, 'being a woman' isn't just about being biologically 'female' in simple sex terms. It is also about living within a social environment where gender relations, expressed for example through **discourses** of 'femininity' and 'masculinity', have a profound effect on women and men's social status, their roles and responsibilities and on their different access to power and material resources.

Sociologists argue that, because social experience is 'gendered' in various ways, there are significant gender divisions in contemporary society. Differences in the experience of health and illness, and in patterns of mortality, are forms of gender division that we'll consider

Keywords

Stereotype
A standardised idea of a person or social group that characterises them, often negatively, in terms of a limited number of 'essential' attributes, behaviours or features.

Keywords

Socialisation
The processes through which people learn the norms and values of society. The outcome is that the individual becomes a socialised member of the society in which they live. Primary socialisation occurs during infancy and childhood. Secondary socialisation continues throughout life as we encounter a wide variety of new social situations and adapt to our changing society.

Discourse
Widely used within sociological literature, generally meaning a way of thinking, or a collection of related statements or events that define relationships between elements of the social world.

more closely later in this chapter. However, in order to understand the social basis of women's health experience, it is necessary to briefly outline the changing contexts of women's lives in contemporary society.

Women's lives in contemporary society

Sociological literature, especially the material focusing on social policy issues, often presents a contrast between a historical 'then' and a contemporary 'now' to show how women's lives have changed over time. Within this type of framework it's possible to illustrate that a woman's life is no longer so closely tied to a housewife/mother role and that significant changes have occurred in patterns of family life and personal relationships during the latter part of the 20th century. While this may be positive in terms of establishing and improving access to equal rights in law, these changes also appear to have led to health consequences for women.

Changing relationships in the family

The nature of the modern family has been affected by a decline in the prevalence of the extended family and an increase in the diversity of family types (Figure 6.1). The changing roles of men and women, both in the family and in wider society, has played a significant part in bringing this about.

The traditional, stereotypical view of male and female roles in the family is that a woman's primary status, and 'duty', is that of housewife and mother. The traditional expectation, widely held until the powerful feminist challenges of the 1960s, was that married women should stay at home to concentrate on 'maternal' tasks such as cooking, cleaning and childbearing. In contrast, men were expected to have a more limited paternal role within the family. The general **social norm** was for men to spend most of their time working in order to provide for the family's needs. As such, men gained most of their status from work roles and the authority position ('head of the household') they held within the home. Until these differing maternal and paternal roles were challenged from the 1960s onwards, they seemed inevitable and 'natural'.

Changing maternal and paternal roles

Gradually the 'traditional' pattern of family roles has changed. Increasingly fathers take on more practical responsibility within

◦━ᴋ Keywords

Social norms

The unspoken and unwritten 'rules' of everyday life in a society. Social norms are learnt through observing others and by noting how other people react to us.

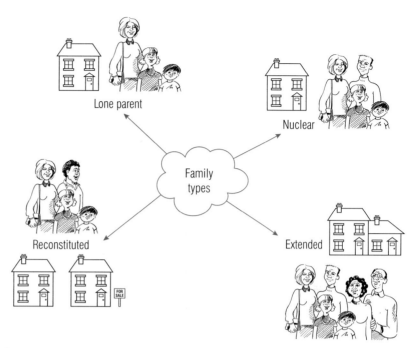

Figure 6.1 *Family types in Britain*

the home and generally make a much greater contribution to child care than in the pre-1960s era, for example. Women have made a lot of progress in terms of gaining greater access to, and equality in, the workplace. However, recent claims that a 'New Man' has emerged who takes on his share of responsibilities within the family are disputed (and not only by academic feminists!).

The recent claims that relationships within the family are now equal because so-called 'New Men' do their share of the practical tasks is disputed and difficult to find hard evidence for. While maternal and paternal roles have converged a great deal since the 1950s, women still seem to actually carry out most of the practical household tasks even though their male partners argue that they 'help'. The primary responsibility for what was seen as the 'maternal' role still appears to lie with women, even though it is accepted that this is no longer a biologically 'natural' role for women, as was previously claimed.

Women's roles in the family gradually changed during the 20th century as a result of a decline in male authority and dominance. Women are no longer expected to play a subservient, supporting role to their male partners and now enjoy greater equality with men in

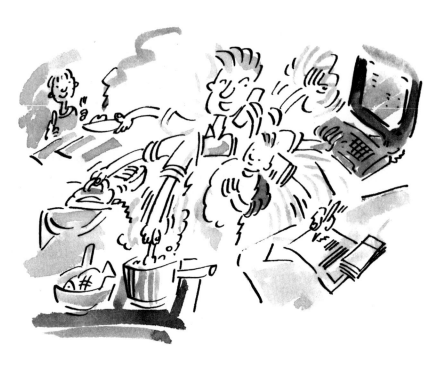

New Man – Modern Myth or Masculine Miracle?

the family and in wider society. Sociological reasons for this include the following:

- **Changes in childbirth patterns**: Women now have fewer children than in the past and are more likely to have them at a later age. This means that women spend less time in child rearing and have more opportunity to establish and develop their careers. A growing number of women are also choosing not to have children at all.

- **An increase in the proportion of women in employment**: This is obviously related to the changing patterns of childbirth but is also due to the increased availability of child care, nursery education and maternity pay. Additionally, the extension of legal rights (equal pay and anti-discrimination) and challenges to cultural expectations about the 'natural' role of women have increased women's access to, and participation in, paid employment.

Patterns of marriage and cohabitation

Fewer people are getting married than 20 years ago. Despite this, most British adults do get married at some point in their life. In

2000 there were 267,961 marriages. However, there were only 156,140 first marriages. The rest were remarriages. There are now fewer first marriages because the average age of first marriage has increased (28 for men, 26 for women) and more people now cohabit, or live together, without marrying. Approximately 10% of adults in Britain are cohabiting at present – this includes 30% of adults under 35 years of age. This doesn't mean that marriage is less popular than it used to be. On the contrary, many people who divorce remarry and many couples who cohabit go on to get married.

Changing patterns of cohabitation and divorce are social trends that illustrate the changing nature of personal relationships and give some indication of the way in which women now have greater social freedom than previously. However, it is important not to jump to the conclusion that women have achieved equality with men, have sexism under control and have broken through all of the old gender barriers that restricted their lives in the past. Large amounts of quantitative and qualitative research evidence are regularly produced by academic sociologists and via the government's own statistics to demonstrate that women do not, in practice, enjoy equality with men. There remains a significant disparity in average levels of pay and in the prevalence of women in positions of power and status in the workforce. Sociologists argue that gender expectations of women still revolve around the issues of reproduction and family responsibility. It seems that it is women, rather than men (New or otherwise) who have to cope with a dual work–family role and all the conflicts and health consequences that this entails.

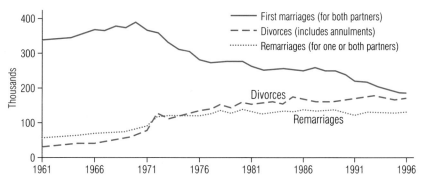

Figure 6.2 *Patterns of marriage and divorce in Britain (redrawn from* Social Trends 29 HMSO)

Gender and caring

Women have access to far greater educational and work opportunities in the 21st century than their mothers and grandmothers enjoyed in the 20th century. Legal rights for women have improved, as have social attitudes towards, and expectations of, women who work outside of the home. While many sociologists, especially feminists, view these changes as evidence of social and political progress for women it is important not to lose sight of a number of negative consequences that also seem to accompany them.

In particular, the persistent association of women with a 'natural' caring disposition and role has led to situations where women are seen as, and are expected to be, unpaid carers within the family regardless of whether they also have employment outside of it.

Paid work and 'careers' are still widely seen as secondary to what is assumed to be a woman's primary role – being the main family carer. Sociological critics argue that the overburdening of women who work arises because there is an unequal distribution of power between men and women in society and unequal access to resources. There is evidence that this has a number of health consequences for such women.

In addition, there is some evidence that the apparent improvement in women's access to employment and resources is still limited by the 'natural carer' stereotype. Where women undertake paid employment outside the home, it tends to be in occupational areas related to 'caring' and personal service. The large-scale employment of women in health, education and social welfare settings is a good example of this. The relative absence of women in the technology and engineering sectors tends to further illustrate the way in which gender expectations lead to and reinforce the occupational segregation of men and women.

> ## Over to you
>
> In what ways do you think that male health-care workers conform to, and differ from, the gender stereotype of men in British society?

Gendered patterns of health and illness

Research studies carried out by academic sociologists, health-care professionals and government bodies provide a wealth of data that reveals persistent differences in patterns of health and illness experience according to gender in Britain.

Patterns of life expectancy and mortality

Death rates for members of both genders have been declining since the mid-19th century. In fact, since 1971 death rates have decreased by 29% for men and by 25% for women. However, the historical pattern of women having a longer life expectancy than men continues to hold true even though the life expectancy gap between the sexes is narrowing.

Cause of death (mortality) varies between the genders. Men are most likely to die from circulatory diseases while the main cause of death for women is now cancer. According to the European Commission (1997), British women are much more likely to die from cancer (42%) than women from other European countries (26%). Breast cancer is the most prevalent cause of death in British women, followed by lung cancer.

The overall pattern of mortality varies between the genders too. For example, while the age-specific mortality rates for males are higher throughout life, they peak at certain ages. In particular, the high-risk period for men is between 15 and 22 with the higher rates of death resulting mainly from motor vehicle accidents. Boys are also far more likely than girls to die from accidents in childhood.

Gendered patterns of morbidity

Gender differences are not so clear when it comes to morbidity. While women do self-report more ill health than men and make more use of health-care services, the reasons for these patterns are not clear. There is, in fact, some doubt and dispute over the popular contention that 'women are sicker but men die quicker'. One of the

Social class	*n*	Very good	Good	Fair	Bad and very bad
Men					
1 and 2	585	43	44	10	2
3N	139	40	41	16	3
3M	456	30	42	23	5
4 and 5	274	29	38	25	8
Women					
1 and 2	598	43	40	15	2
3N	256	35	43	17	5
3M	442	25	43	26	6
4 and 5	382	25	41	26	8
Total	3236				

Table 6.1 Self-reported general health (%) by gender and social class of head of household (data from White *et al.* 1993)

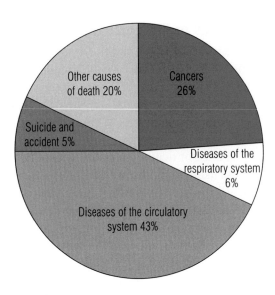

Figure 6.3 *Main causes of death of women in the European Union, 1992 (from The State of Women's Health in the European Community)*

possible reasons for this observation is that sociologists have studied the reporting of illness by women quite closely but have not paid the same attention to men. As such, the apparent statistical pattern may be an artefact, or product, of research processes rather than a real-life phenomenon.

Analysis of patterns of self-reported illness tend to show that, once age is taken into account, there is very little difference in the proportions of men and women reporting limiting, long-standing illnesses. While women are likely to report marginally more illness, as a group they also live longer than men and are therefore more likely to report ill health in their final years.

Explaining gender inequalities in health experience

There does appear to be some statistical evidence of gender inequalities in health experience. However, establishing an empirical pattern isn't the same thing as explaining it. How can these gender patterns be explained? A number of possible explanations have been advanced. Some of these explanations are used by sociological researchers themselves while others are employed as popular, lay explanations or are presented by non-sociological disciplines.

The artefact explanation

This suggests that different gender patterns in morbidity 'exist' because of the way that data are sought and collected rather than because of any real difference in illness experience between men and

Table 6.2 Self-reported health problems by gender (%) (data from OPCS 2002)

Problem	Age range				
	16–44	45–64	65–74	75 and over	All aged 16 and over
Males					
Pain and discomfort	18	39	52	56	32
Mobility	6	22	36	50	18
Anxiety or depression	12	19	20	19	15
Problems performing usual activities	5	16	21	27	12
Problems with self-care	1	6	8	14	5
Females					
Pain and discomfort	20	40	51	65	34
Mobility	6	21	37	60	19
Anxiety or depression	18	24	25	30	22
Problems performing usual activities	7	17	23	40	15
Problems with self-care	2	5	9	21	6

women. For example, morbidity data are collected on the basis of self-reported symptom surveys and statistics compiled from general practitioner (GP) data. One type of artefact explanation suggests that women's morbidity rates are higher because they are culturally conditioned to express their personal health concerns while men are conditioned to conceal their emotions and worries more. The higher rates could therefore reflect women's greater willingness and cultural ability to seek help for and discuss illness symptoms rather than being evidence of higher rates of ill health in women.

One consequence of this is that the official statistics on men's apparently lower morbidity rates may, in fact, be the tip of a male illness 'iceberg'. It has also been pointed out that, as women generally take on responsibility for child care and child health, they are likely to have more contact with general practitioners for family health reasons. A consultation about a child's health may also provide opportunities for, or result in, a discussion of the mother's own health and well-being.

The genetic or biological differences explanation

This explanation locates the explanation for gender differences within male and female bodies. Essentially, the argument is that men and women are vulnerable or predisposed to different kinds of disease and illness 'risk' because of their biological differences. You've probably already noticed that this isn't an explanation that addresses the issue of gender. Rather it conceptualises the problem in terms of sex differences.

Sociologists would criticise this explanation on a number of grounds. Firstly, the notion of genetic or biological differences between men and women overplays the nature and limited extent of innate differences between the sexes. Physiologically and anatomically, men and women have almost everything in common. Arguably, the secondary sexual and reproductive organ differences that do exist are, in themselves, insufficient to account for different patterns of morbidity and mortality. Secondly, genetic explanations individualise and essentialise the causes of ill health and mortality. They locate causation in the individual and neglect the powerful role of social and cultural factors that affect the health chances of particular groups of women in particular ways. In doing so they fail to recognise the gendered nature of health experience.

Despite the above criticisms of the genetic/biological differences explanation of women's health and illness experiences, there is an area in which women do seem to have a biological advantage over men. Women's longer life expectancy appears to be a global phenomenon. It is possible that women have 'longer life genes' than men. These genes may confer a more robust immune system, and therefore greater protection from disease, on women in comparison to men. However, there is insufficient empirical evidence to say that this is anything more than a hypothesis at present.

Structural/materialist explanations

This type of explanation claims a link between the way in which social life is organised and experienced and health outcomes. In particular, the gendering of occupations is seen as a critical factor that influences gendered patterns of health and illness. Specifically, male occupations are seen to place men at greater risk of experiencing workplace injuries and fatal accidents and of exposing them to the harmful effects of industrial processes, toxic chemicals and other damaging substances. The pattern of higher male mortality from accidents and respiratory diseases provides some support for this. However, as the prevalence of female employment rises the entry of women into areas of the workforce that were once the preserve of men may result in a rebalancing of the gendered pattern of work-related health problems. But what if the gendered pattern of work-related morbidity and mortality fails to change? In such circumstances male work culture and men's behaviour in the workplace, in particular their attitudes and responses to hazards and risk, may come to be seen as the key variables underpinning the link between occupation and health experience.

Culture, lifestyle and health behaviour explanation

This explanation has just been touched on. The suggestion is that gendered patterns of risk-taking behaviour account for gendered patterns of health and illness experience. For example, young men are much more likely to die prematurely from road traffic accidents and while participating in dangerous sports than young women. Although aggressive social behaviour is culturally encouraged and approved of in men, the consequence is more male deaths and injuries. Generally, men are also likely to drink more alcohol, smoke more tobacco and are more involved in substance misuse than women. These activities all involve significant health risks. However, if the recent trend of large numbers of young women taking up smoking continues, the gendered pattern of smoking-related diseases is likely to even out.

None of these four approaches provides a wholly satisfactory explanation for gendered patterns of morbidity and mortality. There may, in particular circumstances, be some truth in all of them. However, sociologists who are keen to identify how elements of 'the social' impact on and shape our lives, are most likely to employ versions of the structural/materialist and cultural (lifestyle/health behaviour) explanations. In doing so they tend to draw attention to the way that notions of gender (what it means to be 'masculine' or 'feminine') are implicated in the choices we make, the way we behave and the responses and expectations of other people. For sociologists, gender differences inevitably result in gendered patterns of mortality and morbidity because they establish and maintain the different conditions in which men and women live their lives.

Who is complaining?

One of the interesting, and little commented on, features of the empirical data in this area is that women seem to fare better than men in terms of health experience. Though women of working age (16–64 years) do, on average, report more illness symptoms and consult medical practitioners more often each year than men, this is not evidence that as a population they are actually sicker than men. In fact, premature mortality, the ultimate outcome of ill health, is still a more likely experience for men rather than women. While not wishing to diminish or underplay the significance of women's experience, recent work in this area has finally recognised the need to consider how and why men's experience of health and illness is also gendered.

Reflective activity

Reflect on the ways that you might make use of the concept of 'gender' within your health-care practice. How might your greater awareness of gender issues and processes benefit the people you provide care for as well as yourself?

Rapid recap

Check your progress so far by working through each of the following questions.

1. Define the terms 'sex' and 'gender'.

2. Why, according to sociologists, is it important to distinguish between sex and gender when exploring women's health issues?

3. Describe the ways in which patterns of morbidity and mortality are 'gendered' and outline how these gender patterns can be explained.

If you have difficulty with more than one of the questions, read through the section again to refresh your understanding before moving on.

References

European Commission (1997) *The State of Women's Health in the European Community*. Office for Official Publications of the European Community, Luxembourg.

Office of Population Census and Surveys (OPCS) (2002) *Living in Britain: General household survey*. HMSO, London.

White, A., Nicolaas, G., Foster, K. *et al.* (1993) *Health Survey for England* 1991. HMSO, London.

Further reading

Annandale, E. and Hunt, K. (2000) *Gender Inequalities in Health*. Open University Press, Buckingham.

MacIntyre, S., Hunt, K. and Sweeting, H. (1996) Gender differences in health: are things really as simple as they seem? *Social Science and Medicine*, **42**, 617–624.

Miers, M. (2000) *Gender Issues and Nursing Practice*. Palgrave Macmillan, Basingstoke.

Northrup, C. (1995) *Women's Bodies, Women's Wisdom*. Piatkus, London.

Prior, P. (1999) *Gender and Mental Health*. Macmillan, London.

Wilkinson, S. and Kitzinger, C. (eds.) (1994) *Women and Health: Feminist Perspectives*. Taylor & Francis, London.

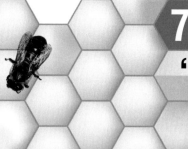

7

'Race', ethnicity and health

Learning outcomes

By the end of this chapter you should be able to:

- Discuss and distinguish between the concepts of 'race', 'ethnicity' and 'ethnic group'
- Describe the difficulties of researching and recording 'ethnic' patterns of health and illness
- Outline patterns of health and illness experience of ethnic groups in Britain
- Apply knowledge and understanding of ethnic patterns of health and illness to health-care practice.

The emergence of 'race' as a concept

The first significant issue that health-care practitioners need to address in this area is the meaning and use of the term 'race'. This is a highly charged and controversial area of popular and academic discourse, not least because the question of whether different human 'races' exist is heavily disputed. The term 'race' is placed in speech marks here to indicate that sociologists invariably contest, and often reject, the term.

Sociologists who criticise and reject the notion of 'race' as a 'natural', scientifically justifiable way of categorising 'types' of people generally argue that 'race' is a socially constructed typology. The concept is said to have its historical origins in 18th and 19th century colonial assumptions about the differences between white and non-white people. Critically, the concept of 'race' is seen as a product of racist value judgements about the 'natural' superiority of 'white' people in comparison to other 'races'.

Michael Banton (1987) distinguishes between three types of 'race' theory:

- **The 'race' as lineage approach**: While we're all viewed as a part of the same evolving human race, this approach suggests that at some point people became differentiated into distinct lines of descent or lineage. The evidence of this is seen in differences in the physical appearance and geographical origin of different groups of people.
- **The 'races' as types of people approach**: This approach argues that, in effect, different 'types' of people have different evolutionary origins that divide human beings into distinctive groups. The popularity of this theory in the 19th century led some medical and social commentators to argue that 'Negro' and 'white' 'races' should not 'amalgamate' and should avoid becoming 'tainted' through interbreeding.

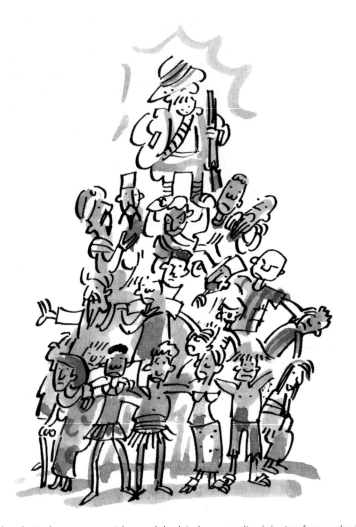

'Race' is rejected as a concept by sociologists because it originates from colonial ideas about the superiority of white people

- **The 'race' as subspecies approach**: This is a combination of the previous two approaches. It originates from the work of Charles Darwin on 'natural selection'. The 'race' as subspecies approach suggests that a number of dominant subspecies of human being have evolved through processes of selection.

All of these approaches accept the notion that biologically distinct 'races' exist within the human population. Sociologists, and many scientists, criticise and reject this basic idea.

Rejecting the biological basis of 'race'

For sociologists, 'race' is best understood as an idea that is historically situated and meaningful in the context of particular political, economic and social relations. Instead of being a 'scientific' reality, 'race' is seen as a concept that derives from, and only makes sense within, particular social conditions and relationships. In particular, sociologists argue that the concept of 'race' was used to make sense of the oppression and domination of non-white people by their white, Western colonisers. In addition to criticising the concept of 'race' on sociopolitical grounds, sociological critics of 'race' sometimes also employ science itself to challenge the idea. They argue that 'race' does not even exist in any meaningful biological way, given that there is more genetic variation within so-called 'racial' groups than there is between them (Jones 1991). On this basis, genetic similarity does not, in itself, define 'race'.

It is important to note that sociologists do recognise that a notion of 'race' is sometimes part of a person's self-defined sense of identity. Where this occurs sociologists refer to *socially defined 'races'* to acknowledge that some ethnic groups perceive themselves and others as having distinct biological characteristics. Regardless of whether this is true in reality, the perception can have an impact on a person's life chances and social experience.

The 'ethnic' alternative

⊶ Keywords

Ethnicity
A sense of identity that is based on shared cultural, religious and traditional factors. Ethnicity can, but does not have to, have a 'racial' dimension.

Within sociology social and cultural factors, rather than biological characteristics, are seen to be of greatest significance when categorising people. '**Ethnicity**' – or 'ethnic origin' – is the alternative term that is used to describe what are seen as social and cultural distinctions between different 'types' of people. However, like 'race', the concept of ethnicity is also far from unproblematic despite its wider use and greater acceptability in both popular and academic discourse.

> ## Over to you
>
> - How do you define your own 'ethnicity'?
> - To what extent is your ethnicity an important part of your sense of identity?

What is an 'ethnic group'?

Sociologists identify an 'ethnic group' as a culturally distinct section of the population. Distinctions can occur between different groups within a population on the basis of language, religion, 'race', ancestral homeland or way of life for example. The perception of difference, and therefore the definition of who belongs to an ethnic

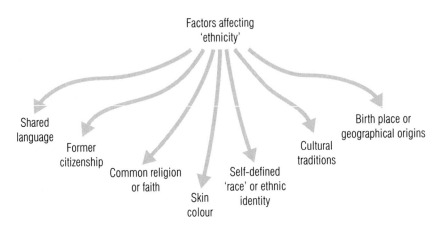

Figure 7.1 *Factors affecting 'ethnicity'*

group, can be made by members of the group themselves or by people outside it.

'Ethnic groups' can be identified in terms of various shared characteristics. For example, people who have a common former citizenship, such as Albanians, West Indians or Ethiopians, can be seen to constitute specific ethnic groups in Britain. Alternatively, an 'ethnic group' may be seen to consist of a subsocietal group that has a common descent and cultural background. For example, Romany gypsies and British 'Italian' people are seen to be ethnically distinctive for this reason. Finally, an 'ethnic group' can consist of pancultural groups with widely differing cultural and social backgrounds who share a similar language, race or religion. 'Asians' are an example of the way this category is used in Britain. People may be identified as 'Asian' despite their apparently different religious affiliations (Hindu, Muslim, Sikh, for example), ancestral homelands (Bangladesh, Pakistan, India), and their diverse languages (Hindi, Punjabi, Bengali) and cultural traditions.

Typically, people define their 'ethnicity' through reference to cultural factors. Sociologically, the concept of **culture** refers to the beliefs and behaviour guidelines that exist in any society. Culture is learned, or transmitted, from one generation to another, through the process of socialisation. Most people will view their own culture as natural and 'normal' and will often not be aware that their beliefs and behaviours are culturally determined.

⊶ᴛ *Keywords*
....

Culture
A concept often used very broadly by sociologists to include the language, values and norms, customs, forms of dress, type of diet, social roles and knowledge and skills that are part of the way of life of a given society.

Multicultural Britain

Britain is a multicultural society. This means that the population of Britain is composed of a number of different ethnic groups which, to varying degrees, have distinctive cultures that play a significant part in their sense of identity, relationships with others and way of life. The contemporary multicultural character of British society is often traced back to migration, or population movement from British 'commonwealth' countries, particularly the Indian subcontinent and the West Indies, during the 1950s and 1960s. However, it is also important to realise that people of African–Caribbean and Asian origin were already present in Britain in the centuries before Britain obtained its colonial Empire between the 16th and 19th centuries. For example, the Roman armies that invaded Britain in the first century AD included many black soldiers. Historical records show that there was a black community of 15,000 people living in Britain by 1715 (Small 1994).

Many of the black people who came to Britain in the 18th and 19th centuries came to work as soldiers, servants and sailors. Some others were brought forcibly and were kept as slaves until slavery was abolished in Britain in 1838. The economic and military needs of Britain have also been important factors influencing patterns of immigration. For example, the end of the First World War and the Second World War saw an increase in the black population in Britain as people from commonwealth countries and America who had fought for Britain settled here. Additionally, Britain received Protestant and Jewish migrants fleeing religious persecution in both Eastern and Western Europe between the 16th and the 20th centuries and Irish migrants fleeing starvation and poverty, particularly between 1820 and 1910. Migration to Britain is a continuing phenomenon that provokes heated political and popular discussion about its desirability. Many of the debates centre on the possible impact of immigration on Britain as a nation and on relations between the diverse ethnic groups and the British population. However, it is also important to note that many members of Britain's minority ethnic groups are not immigrants at all (Table 7.1).

The ethnic minority population of Britain consists of between 4 and 5 million people, depending on which groups are included. For example, the inclusion of Irish people increases the numbers, although in some statistics 'Irish' is assumed to be part of the 'white, British' ethnic category. The age structure of the ethnic minority population is younger than that of the majority white population. One-third of people classed as members of ethnic minorities are under the age of 16, compared to approximately a fifth of the majority white population. At the other end of the age spectrum, a much larger proportion of the white population is made up of older people (aged 65+) compared to the ethnic minority population. As a

Table 7.1 Population of the UK by ethnic group, 2001 (data from ONS 2004)			
	Total population		**Non-white population**
	n	%	(%)
White	**54,153,898**	**92.1**	–
Mixed	**677,117**	**1.2**	**14.6**
Indian	1,053,411	1,8	14.6
Pakistani	747,285	1.3	16.1
Bangladeshi	283,063	0.5	6.1
Other Asian	247,664	0.4	5.3
All Asian or Asian British	**2,331,423**	**4.0**	**50.3**
Black Caribbean	565,876	1.0	12.2
Black African	485,277	0.8	10.5
Black Other	97,585	0.2	2.1
All Black or Black British	**1,148,738**	**2.0**	**24.8**
Chinese	**247,403**	**0.4**	**5.3**
Other ethnic groups	**230,615**	**0.4**	**5.0**
All minority ethnic populations	**4,635,296**	**7.9**	**100.0**
All population	**58,789,194**	**100**	

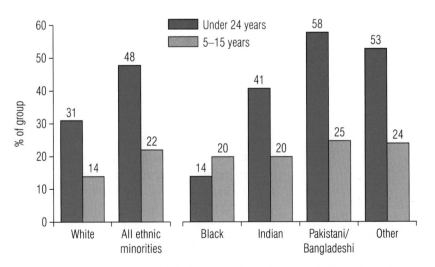

Figure 7.2 *Young people in Britain by age and ethnic group, 1997 (redrawn from Labour Force Survey 1997)*

consequence of this difference in age structure, the ethnic minority population is growing at a faster rate than the white population. Between 1992 and 1999 the ethnic minority population grew by 15.6% compared to a 1% growth in the white population.

Britain's ethnic minority groups are mainly located in large cities and metropolitan areas. Almost half of the total ethnic minority population, particularly African–Caribbean groups, live in London. However, large clusters of people classified as 'ethnic minorities' can also be found in Leicester (Indian) and Bradford (Pakistani), for example. Despite these apparent concentrations, it is also the case that the white majority population in even the most monocultural

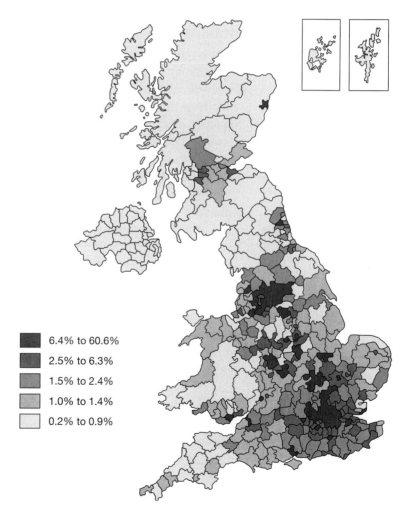

6.4% to 60.6%
2.5% to 6.3%
1.5% to 2.4%
1.0% to 1.4%
0.2% to 0.9%

Figure 7.3 Ethnic diversity throughout Britain (from ONS 2004)

areas of Britain is familiar with the multicultural nature of the broader population, even if they have relatively little direct experience of such groups.

> ## Over to you
>
> - How ethnically diverse is the local population in the area where you live and work?
> - What impact do you think that ethnic diversity has on social relationships within your local area or workplace?

Hostility towards ethnic minorities in Britain

Though multicultural Britain has a long-standing history, most black immigration has occurred since 1945. In the early 1950s, people from the commonwealth nations such as India, Pakistan and the islands of the West Indies, were invited to Britain to work on the reconstruction of Britain's damaged housing, railways, hospitals and factories because indigenous British workers were in short supply. Sir Winston Churchill visited Jamaica in the West Indies and spoke to the 'British subjects' in ringing tones of their 'motherland' and urged them to 'come and rebuild' it. Many of them were skilled, educated workers, such as teachers, nurses and civil servants, who gave up their jobs, homes and families to come to the UK, only to be treated with indifference by members of the indigenous population who were not used to people of a different colour.

However, the problems experienced by members of minority ethnic groups are much greater and more deeply rooted than this alleged 'indifference' of the indigenous population. Active racism and substantial racial discrimination have had a direct impact on the lives of people who belong to ethnic minority groups in Britain since immigration began. In the 1950s and 1960s members of ethnic minority communities suffered a great deal of overt (and at the time lawful) racial discrimination to the point where they experienced difficulties obtaining work and accommodation. This was hardly the welcome they expected from the 'mother country'. Many sociologists and members of ethnic minority groups would argue that racism and racial discrimination are still a significant issue in British society, despite greater awareness and cultural disapproval of it.

Racism and racial discrimination

Racism is a form of **prejudice**. When individuals act on their prejudices they treat the targets of their prejudice in an unfair,

⊶ Keywords

Prejudice
An opinion, feeling or attitude of dislike concerning another individual or group of people. Prejudices are usually unfavourable, unreasonable and unfair judgements that are not based on accurate information or fact and may be held even when proved to be unjustified or false.

unequal way. This is unfair discrimination. Racism is racial prejudice. Acting in a racist way often leads to racial discrimination.

Racism and racial discrimination are based on the belief that one ethnic group of people is naturally superior to other ethnic groups. Racists usually make distinctions between, and judgements about, people on the basis of their physical appearance, particularly the colour of their skin. In Britain, where the majority of the population is white, racism is usually directed against non-white minority ethnic groups. Racist beliefs are used to justify the inferior and unfair treatment of members of minority ethnic groups and to deny members of these groups equality of opportunity.

Racial inequalities are created by, and unfortunately continue to be maintained by, people at all levels within British society. Racism doesn't simply exist on an individual level between people and shouldn't be explained only in terms of individual prejudice. For example, *institutional racism* is said to be expressed through organisational practices, policies and procedures that operate in ways that fail to give people from ethnic minority groups a fair chance or equal treatment and which support 'exclusionary practices'. Institutional racism is a controversial concept because it refers to racism that is covert and hidden and may well be inadvertent. The concept of cultural racism extends this further by suggesting that the indigenous British population is, in fact, culturally conditioned to make sense of ethnic minority cultures in terms of the attributes and capabilities of the 'racial groups' that allegedly constitute them.

The social nature of inequality

People are born with individual differences. However, it is wrong to think that biologically based differences in physical appearance and ability and in mental capacity are the cause of the broad range of inequalities that exist in society. The causes of inequalities in society are social. This means that inequalities (rather than *differences*, remember!) between people result from the ways in which society is divided and structured.

British society is divided and structured according to social class, 'race', gender, disability, age and, to some extent, sexuality. Some people achieve more power and success than others because they are born, or manage to get themselves, into the social groups that have more power and advantages. In British society people who are white, middle-class, male, heterosexual and able-bodied have greater power and opportunities than people who are non-white, working-class, female, homosexual or disabled.

When thinking about the role that care practitioners and care organisations have in promoting equality, remember that discrimination and unfair treatment are closely associated with social or structural inequality. Inequality is not simply the result of individual differences in physical and mental ability, and unfair discrimination involves more than unacceptable behaviour by 'bad' people.

Reflective activity

Reflect on the possible responses that you could make if you witnessed or experienced an incident of racism or racial discrimination in a health-care setting. Does ignoring the racism of a service user or colleague amount to condoning it or are there circumstances in which this is the best response?

Ethnicity and health experience

The social patterning of health and illness experience on 'racial' or ethnic lines is an issue that arouses controversy and is treated with some caution by sociologists. The basis of the controversy in this area centres on the issue of innate or inherited differences between people of different 'races'. In essence, are some people naturally more susceptible to certain diseases and forms of illness because of their 'racial' inheritance and constitutions? As you will no doubt be aware by now, sociologists tend to question and challenge explanations that rely on 'nature' and biology to explain what they see as social patterns of health experience. We will explore this issue in more detail below.

The other major aspect of controversy in this area is whether people who belong to minority 'ethnic' groups in Britain experience particular patterns of mortality, disease and ill health because of the effect of social and cultural factors. It has been argued by sociologists, and many health-care practitioners, that the patterns of health and illness experienced by ethnic minority groups are caused by specific social factors. In particular, members of minority ethnic groups tend to live in poorer social conditions, experience greater stress and hostility (especially through racism) and have lifestyles and cultural practices that increase the risk of ill health. Nevertheless, these claims are contested and the area remains a problematic one to research and obtain reliable data on.

Table 7.2 Standardised mortality ratios for people aged 20–64 years in England and Wales by country of birth, 1991–93 (data from Davey Smith *et al.* 2000)

Ethnic group	All causes	Ischaemic heart disease	Stroke	Lung cancer	Other cancer	Accident and injuries	Suicide
Men							
Caribbean	89	60	169	59	89	121	59
West/South Africa	126	83	315	71	133	75	59
East Africa	124	160	113	37	77	86	75
Indian subcontinent							
India	106	140	140	43	64	97	109
Pakistan	102	163	148	45	62	68	34
Bangladesh	133	184	324	92	74	40	27
Scotland	129	117	111	146	114	177	149
Ireland	135	121	130	157	120	189	135
Women							
Caribbean	104	100	178	32	87	103	49
West/South Africa	142	69	215	69	120	–	102
East Africa	127	130	110	29	98	–	129
Indian subcontinent	99	175	132	34	68	93	115
Scotland	127	127	131	164	106	201	153
Ireland	115	129	118	143	98	160	144

– = no data. 100 = average for the whole population.

Using 'ethnicity' to explore patterns of health and illness experience

Despite the problems of classifying a person's 'ethnicity', sociologists see the concept of 'ethnic group' as the best available way of exploring social patterns of health experience across cultural groups. The concept of 'ethnicity' recognises that social divisions between different cultural groups in the population are identifiable and have an impact on health and well-being. Nevertheless, we still need to be cautious about the basis on which data about ethnicity and health have been compiled.

Many of the early, pioneering studies carried out on 'race' and health experiences were methodologically weak. One reason for this was that researchers often defined 'race' in terms of 'place of birth', leading to significant inaccuracies in data. For example, data relating to black British-born people would not be allocated to the correct 'ethnic group' category if 'place of birth' is used as the criterion for defining 'ethnicity'. Consequently, statistics in these older studies tend to reveal more about the health experience of immigrant populations and much less about that of British-born ethnic groups. It is also important to be aware that 'race' is sometimes assumed to be an independent variable affecting health experience, but sociologists now criticise this concept as a 'social construction'.

Additionally, we need to be aware that aggregate 'race' or 'ethnic group' categories such as 'Asian' tend to conflate a number of factors, such as place of birth, social class, religion and lifestyle. This ignores the possibility that these differences between people who are crudely defined as 'Asian' may have their own specific effects on health and illness experience. These issues, and the varying ways of defining 'race' and 'ethnicity', mean that we need to be cautious when making comparisons between the data and findings of different studies that claim to establish a social patterning of health and illness experience according to ethnicity.

Why study the links between ethnicity and health experience?

Members of 'ethnic minorities' comprise only 6% of the total UK population. This said, members of minority ethnic groups have an equal entitlement to appropriate and effective health-care and treatment services. Sociologists study the social patterning of health and illness according to ethnicity because they are interested in and concerned about the possibility that minority ethnic groups experience social inequality, less favourable treatment and reduced 'life chances' compared to the majority (white) population. Studying the general links between ethnicity and health experience provides 'hard' data that is useful to policy-makers and health service planners and also provides 'evidence' on which to challenge inequality and campaign for improvements. Studies that identify links between ethnicity and patterns of specific health conditions also help clinicians to develop and target treatments in ways that are relevant to members of minority ethnic groups.

Patterns of illness and disease by ethnicity

There are relatively few sociological studies on the general links between ethnicity and health experience. However, epidemiological data does present some evidence of an ethnic patterning of health experience. Findings revealed by epidemiological data include:

- All minority ethnic groups have a shorter life expectancy than the majority white population.

- Members of the white British population experience higher rates of cancer and lung disease than members of minority ethnic groups.
- People belonging to groups from the Indian subcontinent are more likely to die from coronary heart disease than members of other ethnic groups.
- Members of African–Caribbean groups experience high mortality from stroke but low rates of cancer.
- African people have higher rates of high blood pressure and are more likely to die as a result of accidents, violence and tuberculosis than members of other ethnic groups.
- Infant mortality rates are higher for most migrant groups but are highest for Pakistan-born mothers.
- Members of minority ethnic groups rate their personal health in poorer terms than members of the white population.
- Some diseases that have a low overall prevalence in the general population have a specific impact on some minority ethnic groups. Sickle cell disease is an example of this.

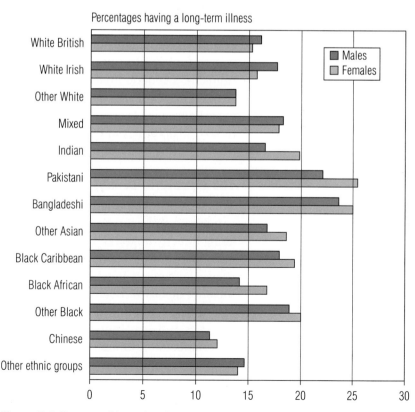

Figure 7.4 *Patterns of long-term illness and disability by ethnicity (from ONS 2004)*

Ways of explaining ethnic patterns of health experience

There are a variety of explanations for the apparent ethnic patterning of health and illness experience in Britain. Some of these explanations are sociological in the sense that they draw on sociological perspectives and identify specific social factors in the causation, or aetiology, of these disease patterns. Other types of explanation attract criticism from sociological thinkers because they claim that 'natural', biological and individualistic factors can account for patterns within a relatively large population of people.

The genetic or biological explanation

The genetic or biological explanation for ethnic patterning of mortality and morbidity is based on the argument that different ethnic groups inherit, or are biologically vulnerable to, certain illnesses and diseases. It does appear to be the case that some disorders have a fundamentally genetic cause that is more prevalent in the ethnic minority population. For example, sickle cell disease is predominant in ethnic West African people because the genetic trait for the disease helps to protect the carrier from malaria. However, genetic inheritance is inadequate as a general explanation for the wider ethnic patterning of morbidity and mortality experience. Arguably, a genetic predisposition to certain disorders only becomes significant when adverse social conditions and negative life experiences, for example, trigger it off. Therefore it is also necessary to take structural and lifestyle factors into account when accounting for the ethnic patterning of morbidity and mortality.

The structural or material factors explanation

This type of explanation points to the material surroundings, living conditions and economic situation that a social group experiences as being directly linked to their 'life chances' and health experience. As such, patterns of health experiences are seen as a consequence of the social context in which minority ethnic groups live. Occupation, income, quality of housing, diet and 'social position' are seen as inter-related and linked to health outcomes. An array of official statistics and academic studies have shown that ethnic minorities experience more unemployment, poorer housing, worse social conditions and higher stress than the indigenous white population. From a structuralist position these experiences are seen to translate into ill health and higher mortality rates. However, while there is a research base to support the general argument made by structuralists, this approach doesn't explain the higher incidence of specific disorders in particular ethnic minority groups or the variation in health experiences between ethnic minority groups or within particular groups. Other explanations do this more convincingly.

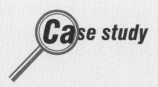

Case study

Cooper, H. (2002) Investigating socio-economic explanations for gender and ethnic inequalities in health. *Social Science and Medicine*, **54**(5), pp. 693–706.

This paper examines inequalities in the self-reported health of men and women from white and ethnic minority groups in the UK. The results show a pattern of substantially poorer health among all minority ethnic groups compared to whites of working age. Ethnic minority women have higher morbidity rates than their male counterparts. This pattern is not repeated in the white population. The analysis found that marked socioeconomic differences were linked to morbidity rates – high morbidity is concentrated in adults who are most socioeconomically disadvantaged. These tended to be people from Bangladeshi and Pakistani backgrounds.

The cultural or individual behaviour explanation

These explanations are often used 'officially' and have become a familiar feature of local and national government health policies and health promotion activity. The suggestion underpinning this type of explanation is that the way of life of a particular ethnic minority group predisposes its members to particular disorders or health problems. A commonly cited example of this is the linking of higher rates of heart disease and rickets in the 'Asian' (especially Indian) population to their dietary intake. The 'unhealthy' behaviour of individuals is also sometimes used in a similar way to explain why some members of ethnic groups and not others experience particular health problems. However, sociological critics tend to criticise this kind of explanation for 'blaming the victim', for ignoring structural factors, such as the effects of poor housing, higher unemployment and lower incomes and for not taking the effects of racism into account.

The racism or unequal treatment explanation

This approach sees 'race' as a critical factor influencing the health and illness experience of minority ethnic groups in Britain. In particular, racial hostility and various forms of discrimination are seen as having an impact on the health experience of the minority ethnic population. For example, the direct personal experience of racism can have an impact on psychological health and well-being as well as an ongoing effect on physical health through increased stress and anxiety. Additionally, people who cite racism and the unequal treatment of minority ethnic groups as a factor determining health experience also point to health services as being institutionally racist and thus failing to meet the health and well-being needs of members of these social groups. If institutional racism is a factor, with services systematically ignoring or failing to deal with the health needs of ethnic minority patients in culturally sensitive ways, the subsequent lack of access to appropriate and effective care will be revealed in higher rates of morbidity and mortality.

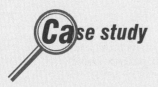
Case study

Karlsen, S. and Nazroo, J. Y. (2002) Agency and structure: the impact of ethnic identity and racism on the health of ethnic minority people. *Sociology of Health and Illness*, **24**(1), pp. 1–20.

This paper argues that, in order to understand ethnic inequalities in health, the relationship between ethnic minority status, structural disadvantage and agency must be explored and worked out. The authors argue that the direct effects of racism on health have so far been ignored in the literature but that there is a relationship between health and experiences of racism, perceived racial discrimination and class.

> ### Over to you
> Find out about the anti-racism policies that are in place in your educational institution or place of work. Are they sufficient to prevent racial discrimination from occurring? Find out how they are monitored and whether there is an adequate complaints and disciplinary process in operation to deal with incidents of racial discrimination.

The artefact explanation

This explanation is used to argue that researchers artificially construct the link between ethnicity and health experience. Some sociologists argue that researchers analysing the ethnic patterning of health are in fact really looking at the effect of social class, not 'race' or ethnicity', on health. They argue that, as members of ethnic minorities are more likely to be in the poorer sections of society, their health and illness experience reflects the effects of this.

None of the approaches outlined above provide a completely satisfactory explanation of the link between ethnicity and health experience. Instead, it is advisable to try and consider how particular patterns of health experience or particular illnesses could be explained by one or more of the available explanations.

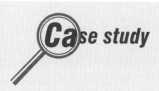
Case study

Nazroo, J. Y. (1998) Genetic, cultural or socio-economic vulnerability? Explaining inequalities in health. *Sociology of Health and Illness*, **20**(5), pp. 710–730.

This study analysed data from a national survey of ethnic minorities to examine three approaches to explaining ethnic inequalities in health. The paper explores the consequences of focusing on ahistoric and de-contextualised genetic and cultural factors at the expense of ignoring the structural disadvantage faced by ethnic minority groups. The study sees wider social inequality as the root cause of health inequality.

Reflective activity

Reflect on your knowledge and understanding of sociological approaches to 'race' and 'ethnicity'. How could you make use of the distinction between the two and your awareness of the ethnic patterning of health and illness experience to provide more culturally sensitive health care for service users?

Rapid recap

Check your progress so far by working through each of the following questions.

1. Explain why the concept of 'race' is contested and usually rejected by sociologists.
2. Define the term 'racism' and explain how 'racial discrimination' is said to involve more than 'bad behaviour' by individuals.
3. Outline three contrasting explanations for the ethnic patterning of health and illness experience in Britain.

If you have difficulty with more than one of the questions, read through the section again to refresh your understanding before moving on.

References

Banton, M. (1987) *Racial Theories*. Cambridge University Press, Cambridge.

Davey-Smith, G., Chaturvedi, N., Harding, S. *et al.* (2000) Ethnic inequalities in health – a review of UK epidemiological evidence. *Critical Public Health*, **10**, 375–407, Taylor and Francis, London. www.tandf.co.uk/journals

Jones, S. (1991) *The Language of the Genes*. Flamingo, London.

Labour Force Survey, 1997.

ONS (2004) Focus on ethnicity. National Statistics Online. Available online at www.statistics.gov.uk/focuson/ethnicity/default.asp.

Small, S. (1994) Black People in Britain. *Sociology Review*, **April**.

Further reading

Ahmad, W. (1993) *'Race' and Health in Contemporary Britain*. Open University Press, Buckingham.

Bhopal, R. (1997) Is research into ethnicity and health racist, unsound or important science? *British Medical Journal*, **314**, 1751.

Fernando, S. (1991) *Mental Health, Race and Culture*. Macmillan Education, Basingstoke.

Mason, D. (1996) Teaching race and ethnicity in sociology. *Ethnic and Racial Studies*, **19**, 782.

8

Understanding illness and behaviour

Learning outcomes

By the end of this chapter you should be able to:

- Identify and describe a number of ways of understanding the definition of 'illness'

- Outline and discuss sociological approaches to understanding illness behaviour and experiences

- Explain how illness can be conceptualised as 'deviance'.

Competing definitions of 'illness'

As we have seen in the previous chapters, sociologists do not take the concepts of 'health', 'disease' and 'illness' for granted. The sceptical approach that results from applying a sociological imagination in health-care settings leads to these concepts being problematised. That is, the 'natural', apparently self-evident meanings of 'health' and 'illness' that are commonly taken for granted in popular and professional 'health' discourses are called into question by sociological thinkers. In this chapter we will consider how the application of sociological concepts and theoretical traditions can be used to define, understand and analyse the experience of 'illness' in a variety of different ways. However, before we can apply our sceptical sociological thinking to 'illness experience' we need to outline and consider how the term is typically defined and used in both health-care and popular, everyday situations.

Medicine and 'illness'

What is the difference between 'illness' and 'disease'? Eisenberg (1977) distinguishes between these concepts by saying that 'patients suffer "illnesses"; physicians diagnose and treat "disease" . . . illnesses are experienced as disvalued changes in states of being and social function: diseases are abnormalities in the structure and function of body organs and systems'. Helman (1981, p. 544) puts it as clearly but slightly differently when saying that 'disease is something that an organ has: illness is something a man has'. What both of these explanations are doing is highlighting the difference between the objective way that 'disease' is diagnosed and the subjective way that 'illness' is identified.

'Illness' is more problematic for the biomedical model than 'disease' precisely because it refers to the subjective experience of 'ill health' or 'unwellness'. Its existence is 'felt' in terms of symptoms but can't be observed as clinical signs or changes that would allow an objective diagnosis to be made. As a consequence, medical practitioners tend to rely on the self-reporting of symptoms by patients when making 'illness' diagnoses. Sometimes these symptoms may be the consequence of a pre-existing 'disease'. At other times they can result from a sense of lower or impaired functioning – feeling 'rough' or 'under the weather', to use common expressions.

Over to you

- Identify an example of a recent 'illness' that you've experienced but did not seek treatment for.
- How could you describe and explain this experience of illness in non-medical terms?

The social nature of illness

Because 'illness' is about how a person feels, it is culturally valued as being a less important indicator of 'health' problems than 'disease'. This last point alludes to the basically *social* nature of illness. The meaning of 'illness', that is what counts (legitimately) as 'illness', is determined by the cultural context in which it occurs. Definitions of illness rely on social definitions of 'normality' (and therefore 'abnormality') and are much more problematic for doctors to pronounce on or determine. Popular definitions of 'illness' that are used in everyday situations by members of the public sometimes coincide with medical definitions of biological 'normality' but sometimes they don't. The important point to note is that 'illnesses' are culturally specific. 'Members of the public' as we've just called people, belong to diverse cultural groups and don't all share the same cultural heritage. As a result people define themselves as 'ill' in different ways, even within the same culture and social group.

Why do popular definitions of 'ill health' matter?

Professional and academic definitions of the concept of 'ill health' don't necessarily chime with the definitions that service users employ in their own lives. Understanding the nature and use of popular, or lay, definitions of 'illness' is important for health-care workers for a number of reasons.

Firstly, popular definitions of 'illness' strongly influence and guide the help-seeking behaviour of service users. This is important with respect to what doesn't count as 'illness' as much as what does. Failure to recognise their symptoms and define them as evidence of ill health can lead people to ignore treatable health problems that may affect the quality, and even the length, of their lives. Secondly, health-care workers who use a medical model approach to 'health' and 'illness' depend to a large extent on their patients identifying the things that they experience or feel as symptoms of ill health. The health-care worker then looks for signs of specific diseases or illness conditions that match or corroborate the patient's symptoms. The key point is that for this type of health-care encounter to occur the patient must either be operating with concepts of 'health' and 'illness' that are compatible with those of the health carer or the health carer must be alert and sensitive to the ways these concepts are identified, defined and applied in popular discourse. It is also possible, and actually common, for different people to interpret and choose to act (or not to act) upon their symptoms in different ways – because they use and employ concepts of 'health' and 'illness' differently.

Sociologists argue that popular definitions of ill health are the product of specific social, cultural, political and economic circumstances and arrangements. An appreciation of the nature and variety of popular beliefs about 'health' and 'illness' will enhance a health worker's understanding of what sociologists refer to as 'illness behaviour'.

> ## Over to you
>
> Approximately one-third of consultations with GPs in Britain involve people who are experiencing some form of emotional or mental health difficulty. Many of the people who experience such problems initially tell the GP about related physical symptoms such as loss of appetite, loss of energy or a poor sleep pattern and are reluctant to refer to any underlying psychological or emotional causes. How would an awareness of this cultural pattern of behaviour help a GP in such a consultation?

Popular approaches to understanding 'illness'

As we've seen, 'illness' refers to the experiential aspects of bodily and mental 'disorder'. It is defined subjectively. These subjective definitions are seen by sociologists to be the products of society and cultural background. A number of sociological studies have identified the way popular definitions of illness distinguish between 'normal' and 'real' illness (Cornwell 1984 and Blaxter and Paterson 1982, for example). 'Normal' illness, which people tend to accept and do not consult health-care workers about, includes what people see as 'wear and tear' problems. These are more often associated with the ageing process, with work roles or with specific 'women's problems' than with ill health. In popular terms, they are often seen as an inevitable, unavoidable part of life. Another common feature of popular ideas about 'illness' is that people often think that its effects can be reduced or minimised by a positive, stoic attitude. This is a kind of 'mind over matter' approach that implies that those with stronger characters are somehow less likely to experience illness or suffer its effects for long.

How do people think about 'illness'?

Chrisman (1977) identified four basic 'logics' of illness and disease that are used in popular discourse:

- **A logic of invasion**. This cites germ theory and other material intrusions as causal agents in the development of illness and disease.
- **A logic of degeneration**. This interprets illness as a consequence of the running down of the body.
- **A mechanical logic**. This sees illness as the result of damage to, or blockages in, bodily structures.
- **A logic of balance**. This sees illness as the outcome of a disruption of harmony between parts of the body or between the individual and the environment.

Blaxter (1983) identified 12 categories of illness causation in her study of middle-aged, working-class Scottish women. The most frequently cited causes were infection, heredity and then environmental factors (such as working conditions).

Pill and Stott (1986) studied working-class mothers and found that they frequently explained short-term, acute illnesses in terms of medical model causes such as viruses, bugs and germs. The experience of these women as recent mothers of young children may have precluded them from citing degenerative and age-related causes.

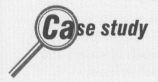
Case study

Lowton, K and Gabe, J. (2003) Life on a slippery slope: perceptions of health in adults with cystic fibrosis. *Sociology of Health and Illness*, **25**(4), pp. 289–319.

This study explored how adults with cystic fibrosis (CF) attending a specialist CF centre perceived their health. CF is traditionally seen as a fatal childhood condition but average survival age is rising. The study showed that adults had varying perceptions of health that were related to the effects of CF, its treatment and the context in which the adults were placed. The study identified four concepts of health – as 'normal', controllable, distressing and a release – that were accompanied by certain coping styles.

The way that people think about and explain their 'illness' experience is, from a sociological perspective, a reflection of their cultural and social experience within a particular society. This explains, for example, why social class differences exist in explanations of 'illness'. People who have a middle-class background tend to believe that they are more able to control their life circumstances and therefore avoid some of the factors that lead to illness. This is in contrast to people with a working-class background, who are likely to be more fatalistic about the risk of becoming 'ill' (see Pill and Stott 1986 and Blaxter and Patterson 1982, for example). The apparent social class differences in the way that people view their ability to control the circumstances that lead to 'illness' may also reflect real differences in the structural pressures and constraints that affect our lives. Middle-class people may be able to exert more control or 'agency' over their everyday life experiences than working-class people because, in structural terms, they have greater freedom to act or are better 'positioned' structurally. In effect, it is harder to avoid 'illness' if you have fewer resources and live in poorer physical circumstances.

Theory Into Practice

Sociological thinking encourages us to consider how a person's social background and cultural viewpoint influence the way in which they define 'health', 'illness' and 'disease', and how they respond to experiences of 'ill health'. This sociological point obviously has important implications for health-care practitioners who seek to provide individualised care that is respectful of and sensitive to a client's values, beliefs and sense of identity.

Exploring illness behaviour

Sociological and epidemiological surveys indicate that people experience a lot of self-defined 'illness' (Figure 8.1). Despite this, most people don't consult medical or other health-care workers with their 'illness' complaints. Health-care practitioners and academics who are interested in this phenomenon, which is often called 'illness behaviour', have tried to explore the different factors that motivate some people to seek professional help while others with the same symptoms don't (and even actively avoid doing so). Sociological approaches to illness behaviour tend to focus on the role that culture and socialisation play in influencing our beliefs about 'health' and 'illness' and on what is referred to as a 'social process' of becoming ill.

The social process of becoming ill

For many sociological thinkers, 'becoming ill' isn't a straightforward, natural or purely biological process. Instead, they argue, a person has to follow a significant social process in order to become 'ill'. Firstly, the person must be able to make a socially appropriate interpretation of their physical and/or mental experiences. That is, they must know what counts as 'illness' within their social world.

The ability to identify physical and mental experiences as symptoms of 'illness' is learnt from a variety of sources, which include family members and friends (as a part of socialisation), the media, educational experiences and experience of using health services. Self-definition of illness relies on the individual being able to use their cultural understanding of 'illness' to make a judgement

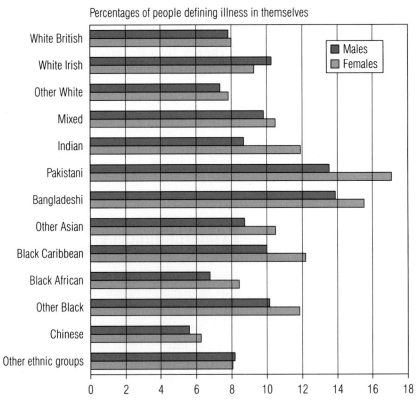

Figure 8.1 *Patterns of self-defined illness (from ONS 2004)*

about whether their bodily or mental experiences are 'normal'. For example, many people expect to feel aches and pains occasionally and have the odd headache. As a result, people often explain such 'felt' symptoms in non-medical ways and accept them as a short-term 'normal' inconvenience.

To progress from a self-defined status of 'normal' inconvenience to being accepted as 'ill', a person's 'felt' symptoms must be recognised by themselves or others as 'abnormal' in some way. Part of the recognition process involves the apparently 'abnormal' experiences being officially acknowledged or legitimised by a health professional or another person, such as a relative or employer, who has the power to confer 'illness' status on them. If you've ever 'phoned in sick' for work or college, you may already have experienced the formalised, bureaucratic procedures that employers use to create 'illness' in this way. Employees or students who don't follow the correct organisational procedures are not, officially, 'ill' and may risk disciplinary action or being recorded as 'absent' instead.

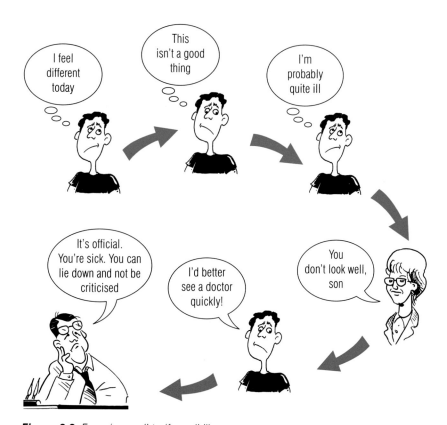

Figure 8.2 *From 'normal' to 'formal' illness*

Irving Zola (1973) is the sociologist credited with developing the concept of a 'social process' of becoming ill. His basic idea is that a person's decision to seek medical help for a perceived 'illness' is a social one that involves consulting other people (family, friends, colleagues) and responding, in part, to their perceptions of the 'health' problem. It is through this process that 'illness' symptoms acquire their meaning. Social interactions with, and pressure from, family and friends are more likely to precipitate a trip to the doctor to have 'illness' confirmed than the severity of a person's symptoms. The significance of a person's symptoms is not always self-evident to the person suffering them. Instead, sociologists argue, people tend to react to the sociocultural meaning that can be attributed to the symptoms by themselves and their significant others.

The personal and social consequences of 'illness'

Early sociological approaches to illness experience tended to address the issue indirectly through theories such as the sick role, labelling theory and work on stigma. Contemporary sociology has a more direct approach to illness experience, focusing on the lived experience of chronic illness. As a result, health-care practitioners and academics now tend to use approaches and concepts drawn from **interactionist** perspectives to understand the meaning, impact and consequences that 'illness' can have on people's lives. Before considering this approach, we will first explore how the concept of the 'sick role' can help us to understand illness behaviour. Unusually this concept does not draw on interactionist sociology but it is useful as a way of understanding how we expect people who acquire an 'illness' status to respond to this.

The sick role

The sociological view of 'illness' as a social state isn't an attempt to deny the personal experience of pain, discomfort or distress that some people suffer or to suggest that there is no biological basis to 'illness' at all. Instead, Talcott Parsons (1951), an American sociologist, sought to identify how our cultural expectations of what it means to be 'ill' determine how we expect people in this state to behave. He argued that in Western societies we expect people to conform to a 'sick role'. Parsons (1951) outlined four components of the 'sick role':

- The sick role legitimately allows social withdrawal and suspension of a person's usual social role obligations – such as going to work or college

○━┭ *Keywords*

Interactionism
An approach to sociological thinking that incorporates a variety of sociological perspectives. The common feature of these perspectives is that they focus on social interaction in everyday life and the meanings that people give to their social experiences and behaviours.

- The legitimately sick person is not held to be responsible for their condition
- The sick person is supposed to find the state of being 'sick' undesirable
- The sick role places a social obligation on the sick person to try to get better by using available health-care resources. Therefore the 'sick' person should not seek to take advantage of the benefits of the sick role (see the first two points).

The concept of the sick role is useful for understanding how society expects people who are 'ill' to behave. It doesn't necessarily help us to understand how people who experience 'illness' actually respond to it. This issue is more directly addressed through the concept of 'biographical disruption' (see below).

Over to you

- Do you think that health-care practitioners use the 'sick role' concept in their care practice?
- You might like to reflect on the links between the concept of the sick role and ideas about 'good' and 'bad' patients in your area of health-care work.

Criticisms of the 'sick role' concept

While the concept of the 'sick role' cannot be criticised for not explaining how people who are 'ill' behave (because it was never intended to), it has been criticised on a range of other grounds. For example, Parsons' (1951) notion of the 'sick role' appears to assume that everyone has equal access to the 'sick role'. However, it is clear that, regardless of the problems they face, some people (especially women within families) do not have the option of withdrawing into the sick role. Additionally, there are some occupational and class-based subcultures where adopting the 'sick role' is not viewed positively but rather as a form of personal and moral 'weakness'.

Critics of the 'sick role' also argue that it fails to take into account situations where a sick person is unwilling to adopt or accept the expectations of the 'sick role' because their 'illness' or condition is socially stigmatised or frowned upon. For example, in situations where people develop epilepsy or a mental disorder, or contract an infectious disease, they may avoid being open about this because these conditions carry a social stigma. Additionally, even when the individual who is suffering a particular condition accepts this and seeks to adopt the sick role, employers, partners or other family members may be reluctant to accept and allow this to happen. This is seen in situations where relatives deny the 'reality' of a family member's clinical diagnosis or illness complaint by disputing the medical basis on which it is made. It is also not uncommon, for example, for employers to resist or dispute complaints of 'stress-related illness' that are made by their employees.

However, despite criticisms of the concept of the 'sick role', it remains a useful way of getting us to think about how society assigns roles and responds to people who claim 'illness'. The moral aspect of 'sick role' judgements is especially pertinent for health carers.

Exploring the experience of illness

The concept of the sick role is useful for understanding how expectations of people who are defined as 'ill' or who seek 'illness' status are essentially social. Since the emergence of the concept of the 'sick role', health-care practitioners and academics have sought to extend our understanding of illness experience by exploring the impact that it has on people's lives and identities. Many of these studies have focused on the experience and impact of chronic illness and have employed a social interactionist approach to do so.

Sociological studies of chronic illness experience have drawn attention to:

- **Uncertainty**: Many chronic conditions have a long, slow onset. During the pre-diagnosis period uncertainty about the meaning and significance of symptoms because of a lack of 'official' recognition through diagnosis can be a source of considerable stress for the individual and their family. Diagnosis can be a welcome relief for many people, even where this in itself does not offer an optimistic picture of the likely course and outcome of the condition. Uncertainty about the day-to-day severity of symptoms can also be a source of stress and disruption to everyday life.

- **Family relations**: The practical and emotional demands of caring for a person with a chronic condition can have a significantly negative impact on marital and family relationships. This is particularly the case if the person experiences pain and other symptoms that are distressing for their partner or wider family to witness. Additionally, the symptoms or treatment after-effects of chronic conditions (such as colostomy surgery) can cause the person to experience shame and embarrassment to a degree that affects their relationships with others.

- **Biographical disruption**: Chronic health problems and disabling conditions have the potential to threaten a person's sense of identity and self-esteem. Bury (1982) developed the concept of 'biographical disruption' to describe the impact that chronic illness experience can have on a person's life. In essence, chronic illness is seen to cause 'biographical disruption' by affecting the expected and planned 'narrative' of a person's life. It requires a rethinking of both the person's biography and their self-concept. This can have both positive (a new direction and re-evaluated sense of self) or negative (a sense of 'loss' of self, threat and lowered self-esteem) consequences.

Williams (1984) extended Bury's (1982) work on 'biography' by arguing that people who experience chronic illness become involved in a process of 'narrative reconstruction'. That is, they reinterpret and retell their life story or biography in light of the onset, and their experience, of the chronic condition or illness. The explanation that the person develops for the onset of their condition isn't necessarily a biomedical one. Rather, it is one that serves the purpose of giving their current and future life experience a sense of meaning and order.

The experience of illness is an area of health-care practice that sociology has been particularly productive in exploring. Caring for people with chronic illnesses is also an area in which non-medical health-care practitioners play a particularly important role. Drawing on the insights of sociology should enable such practitioners to identify, and respond more effectively to, the significant social and emotional needs of people who have chronic illnesses.

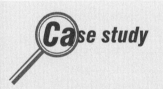

Case study

Sanders, C., Donovan, J. and Dieppe, P. (2002) The significance and consequences of having painful and disabled joints in older age: co-existing accounts of normal and disrupted biographies. *Sociology of Health and Illness*, **24**(2) pp. 227–253.

This study examined the meanings of symptoms for 27 older people aged 51 to 91 years of age with osteoarthritis. The study found that the older participants were most likely to see their symptoms as a normal and integral part of their biography. Younger people were more likely to see their symptoms as significant indicators of 'illness'. All participants were concerned with the disruptive impact that their symptoms had on their daily lives.

Reflective activity

1. Reflect on your understanding of the ways that 'illness' can be explained and is experienced.
2. Do you currently seek and take account of service users' ideas and experiences of 'illness' when planning and delivering care for them?
3. How can you find out about and incorporate service users' own explanations and experiences within your health-care practice?

Viewing 'illness' as deviance

Health-care practitioners and academics who employ interactionist approaches to the definition and understanding of 'illness' argue that illness can be seen as a form of social deviance. Within sociological literature, the term 'deviance' is used to refer to forms of behaviour that break the dominant rules and norms of society. Deviant behaviour isn't always unlawful behaviour. However, it is behaviour that is widely or commonly disapproved of within a specific society and is likely to attract social 'sanctions' or punishment. In a general way, 'illness' can be seen as a form of deviant behaviour because it departs from cultural norms and expectations.

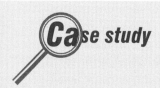 **Case study**

Coyle, J. and MacWhannell, D. (2002) The importance of 'morality' in the social construction of suicide in Scottish newspapers. *Sociology of Health and Illness*, **24**(6) pp. 689–713.

This study examined the reporting of suicide in two broadsheet and two tabloid newspapers in Scotland. The authors argue that reporting sought to make suicide explicable through using concepts of deviancy, dysfunction and moral weakness. The authors argue that the core explanatory category in such stories is 'morality'.

Parsons's (1951) concept of the 'sick role', described earlier, shows how people who are legitimately defined as being 'ill' are allowed to deviate from social norms of 'health'. People in this position are absolved from the general sanctions applied to those who deviate from social norms, because they have gained medical or 'official' (and therefore cultural) approval to withdraw from their normal roles and obligations. Importantly, those who adopt the 'sick role' must submit to medical regulation (which in sociological terms is seen as a form of social control) and be committed to getting better, in order to differentiate themselves from those defined and disapproved of culturally as 'malingerers' and 'hypochondriacs'.

Labelling theory and illness

Health professionals and academics who argue that 'illness' can be understood as a form of social deviance have tended to use labelling theory to develop their arguments. Labelling theory originated in the work of sociologists studying the links between crime and deviance. The main argument of labelling theorists is that definitions of deviance are culturally negotiated during processes of social interaction. 'Deviance' isn't seen as a quality or characteristic of the person or even of the person's behaviour or the act that they carry out. Instead, 'deviance' is seen as a cultural label, containing a strong moral evaluation, that is successfully applied to particular behaviours.

Within a particular society and cultural context, at a particular point or period of history, certain behaviours are defined as 'deviant'. In this sense, 'deviance' labels are socially and culturally relative and historically changeable. This is interesting and useful for health-care workers because there is evidence that a range of behaviours and conditions that are defined in 'illness' terms also have a dual 'deviance' label.

This is particularly the case, for example, with forms of mental illness, substance misuse and so-called 'personality disorder'. Each of these is an 'illness' condition that is defined and labelled at a point of intersection between the discourses of 'health' and

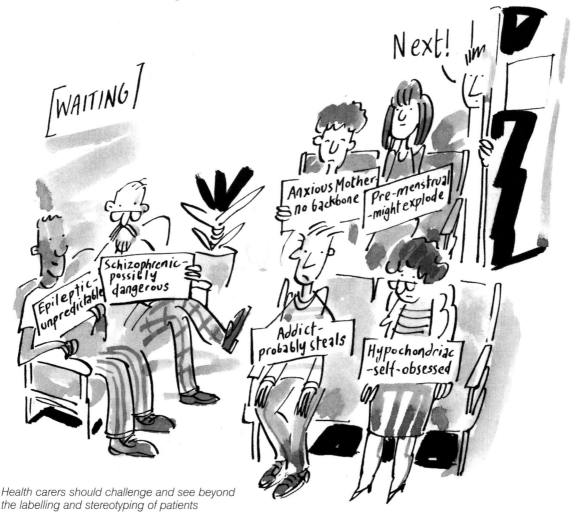

Health carers should challenge and see beyond the labelling and stereotyping of patients

'criminality'. A person medically diagnosed with any of these conditions is also likely to be culturally labelled as 'deviant' by a significant proportion of people in society.

Social stigma and illness

The labelling of 'illness' states as 'deviant' can lead to both psychological and practical problems for people who acquire them. The factor that links the 'deviant' label and these subsequent problems is social stigma.

Social stigma is a concept that refers to the discrediting, devaluation or 'spoiling' of a person's social identity. Essentially, people who suffer some form of social stigma acquire an 'undesired differentness' that taints and reduces them in the eyes of others. Researchers using labelling theory have outlined how social stigma has a significant impact on the lives of those who are diagnosed (i.e. labelled) as 'epileptic' (Scambler and Hopkins 1986, Scambler 1989), with HIV/AIDS (Alonzo and Reynolds 1995, Lawless *et al.* 1996) and suffering from 'mental illness' (Link and Cullen 1983, Hall *et al.* 1993).

People who acquire, or are at risk of acquiring, an illness diagnosis that is stigmatised can find the social stigma more difficult to cope with than the condition itself. Sociologists have developed a number of explanations of how people react to, and try to cope with, the social stigma associated with stigmatising illness labels. For example, Erving Goffman (1968) distinguished between conditions, illnesses or impairments that are *discrediting* and those that are *discreditable*. Where a person's stigmatised condition, illness or impairment is visible and affects their social interaction with others, Goffman argued that it acts as a discrediting attribute. People can see that the person is different in some way and, acting according to dominant beliefs and values, react negatively towards this culturally defined 'abnormality'. In response, people with discrediting attributes often try to use 'impression management' strategies. These seek to avoid, challenge and/or overcome the negative stereotypes and devalued identities that are associated with particular 'illness' labels.

> ## Over to you
>
> - Make a list of illnesses, impairments and conditions relevant to your area of health-care practice that are potentially 'discrediting'.
> - Identify examples of 'impression management' that people who experience such conditions use to avoid becoming labelled as 'abnormal'.

Goffman suggests that, where a person's condition, illness or impairment is invisible, they have the option of trying to keep it a secret. Because 'hidden' or invisible illness labels are only potentially discrediting, the main challenge for people who are subject to them is one of 'information management'.

Scambler and Hopkins (1986) carried out a study of the reactions of people to a diagnosis of 'epilepsy'. Extending Goffman's work on the strategies open to people with stigmatising conditions they explored and theorised about the personal impact that the diagnosis had on people living with this label. They proposed that, while people often challenged the socially stigmatising label of 'epileptic', they still experienced 'hidden distress'. Scambler and Hopkins (1986) argued that 'hidden distress' results from a fear of *enacted stigma* and a sense of *felt stigma*. Enacted stigma occurs where a person publicly experiences prejudice and discrimination because of their 'epilepsy'/'epileptic' labels. Felt stigma occurs where the person experiences the social shame of being labelled 'epileptic' and also fears the occurrence of enacted stigma should their diagnosis be revealed to others. As a result their social identity, behaviour and view of the world are shaped and coloured by the effects (actual and potential) of social stigma.

In a study of people diagnosed with HIV, Alonzo and Reynolds (1995) proposed that participants also experienced a 'stigma trajectory' alongside their 'illness trajectory'. That is, the nature and degree of stigma attributed to, and experienced by, people who are HIV-positive changes over the course of the illness. Alonzo and Reynolds (1995) outlined four phases of the stigma trajectory:

1. **At risk**: This occurs prior to diagnosis and is characterised by uncertainty. The possibility of an HIV-positive diagnosis causes people to experience a 'potentially felt stigma'. There are a variety of responses to this, including denial and the rejection of 'risk'.

2. **Diagnostic**: 'Information management' is the key issue at this stage. Who should be told about the stigmatised diagnosis? 'Felt stigma' is likely to occur here.

3. **Latent**: The individual can conceal their diagnosis and illness condition for a certain amount of time while asymptomatic. Felt stigma is likely but enacted stigma can be avoided during this phase of the illness and stigma trajectories.

4. **Manifest**: 'Deviant' status can no longer be concealed when signs and symptoms of the person's HIV illness become obvious. The person is now more likely to experience enacted stigma at this point in their illness trajectory.

Alonzo and Reynolds's (1995) conceptualisation of the 'stigma trajectory' is useful for showing how the impact of social stigma can vary during a person's illness experience.

Reflective activity

Reflect on your own experiences of providing and receiving health-care services.

To what extent do you think the concepts of 'deviance', 'labelling' and 'stigma' are useful for helping you to understand your own reactions to patients or other people's reactions to your experience of ill health?

How might an awareness of these concepts help health workers to provide care that is more sensitive, supportive and appropriate to the needs of stigmatised service users?

Rapid recap

Check your progress so far by working through each of the following questions.

1. Identify three popular ways of explaining the causes of 'illness'.
2. Describe what happens during the 'social process' of becoming ill.
3. Explain how the concepts of 'deviance', 'labelling' and 'stigma' can be used to understand social responses to certain forms of 'illness'.

If you have difficulty with more than one of the questions, read through the section again to refresh your understanding before moving on.

References

Alonzo, A. A. and Reynolds, N. R. (1995) Stigma, HIV and AIDS: an exploration and elaboration of a stigma trajectory. *Social Science and Medicine*, **41**, 303–315.

Blaxter, M. (1983) The causes of disease: women talking. *Social Science and Medicine*, **17**, 56–69.

Blaxter, M. and Paterson, E. (1982) *Mother and Daughters: a Three Generational Study of Health Attitudes and Behaviour*. London: Heinemann Educational Books.

Bury, M. (1982) Chronic illness as biographical disruption. *Sociology of Health and Illness*, **4**, 167–182.

Chrisman, N. J. (1977) The health-seeking process: an approach to the natural history of illness. *Culture, Medicine and Psychiatry*, **1**, 351–377.

Cornwell, J. (1984) *Hard-earned Lives: Accounts of Health and Illness from East London*. Tavistock, London.

Eisenberg, L. (1977) Disease and illness: distinctions betweeen professional and popular ideas of sickness. *Culture, Medicine and Psychiatry*, **1**, 9–23.

Goffman, E. (1968) *Stigma: Notes on the Management of Spoiled Identity*. Harmondsworth, Penguin.

Hall, P., Brockington, I., Levings, J. and Murphy, C. (1993) Comparison of the responses to the mentally ill in two communities. *British Journal of Psychiatry*, **162**, 99–108.

Helman, C (1981) Disease versus illness in general practice. *Journal of the Royal College of General Practitioners*, **31**, 548–552.

Lawless, S., Kippax, S. and Crawford, J. (1996) Dirty, diseased and undeserving: the position of HIV positive women. *Social Science and Medicine*, **43**, 1371–1377.

Link, B. G. and Cullen, F. T. (1983) Reconsidering the social rejection of ex-mental patients: levels of attitudinal response. *American Journal of Community Psychology*, **11**, 261–273.

ONS (2004) Focus on ethnicity. National Statistics Online. Available online at www.statistics.gov.uk/cci.

Parsons, T. (1951) *The Social System*. Free Press, Glencoe, IL.

Pill, R. and Stott, N. C. H. (1986) Concepts of illness causation and responsibility: some preliminary data from a sample of working-class mothers, in *Concepts of Health, Illness and Disease: a Comparative Perspective* (eds C. Currer and M. Stacey). Berg, Leamington Spa.

Scambler, G. (1989) *Epilepsy*. Routledge, London.

Scambler, G. and Hopkins, A. (1986) Being epileptic: coming to terms with stigma. *Sociology of Health and Illness*, **8**, 26–43.

Williams, G. (1984) The genesis of chronic illness: narrative reconstruction. *Society, Health and Illness*, **6**, 175–200.

Zola, I. K. (1973) Pathways to the doctor – from person to patient. *Social Science and Medicine*, **7**, 677–689.

Further reading

Watt, B. (1996) *Patient – The Story of a Rare Illness*. Viking Books, London.

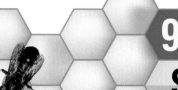

9

Sociology and the body

Learning outcomes

By the end of this chapter you should be able to:

- Understand how the human body can be analysed as a social entity

- Describe sociological approaches to the human body

- Analyse the effects that health-care practices can have on a service user's perceptions and experiences of their body.

Analysing the human body sociologically

Health-care practitioners work very closely with human bodies. There are, in fact, a whole variety of circumstances in which service users quite literally place their bodies in the hands of health-care practitioners. Those who subscribe to and use a biomedical model in their care practice often see 'health', 'illness' and 'disease' as residing, almost by definition, within the human body. We have seen that many medical practitioners also base their work around a conception of the 'normal' body. But, thinking sociologically, can we accept that there is such a thing as the 'normal' body? Being sceptical about taken-for-granted assumptions, we obviously need to subject this idea to more critical sociological analysis.

Sociology has only recently discovered the human body. For a long time, sociologists, like other members of society, viewed the human body as a 'natural' biological entity that had little to do with their research or theoretical agendas. Sociologists are, after all, interested in social structures, processes and practices. The human body seems to have little to do with these aspects of 'the social' world. However, at the beginning of the 21st century there is widespread popular and academic interest in the ways in which the human body is a socially constructed, as well as a 'natural', entity.

The human body as a social entity

The human body is increasingly becoming a focus for sociological analysis because it is being seen as an important 'site' of social meaning and political struggle. Sociologists now argue and seek to show that our understanding of the human body is given 'meaning', or only makes sense, in the context of our awareness and application of discourses of social class, gender, age, 'race' and disability, for example. In this way, the status, and our cultural perception, of the human body is increasingly seen as socially produced or constructed. This doesn't mean that the biological basis of the human body is denied by sociological thinking. Rather, sociological thinking about the human body draws our attention to the ways that people now view their own and other people's bodies as a feature, or expression, of their identity.

Many people dress, develop their physical appearance and use their bodies in ways that consciously express their sense of 'self'. It is increasingly common for people to physically alter their body, through surgery, forms of adornment (tattooing and piercing, for example) or fitness training, in order to achieve an ideal, or at least a preferable, self-image. As a result, the human body can be sociologically analysed as a site of social meaning, or what Featherstone *et al.* (1991) call 'the visible carrier of the self'.

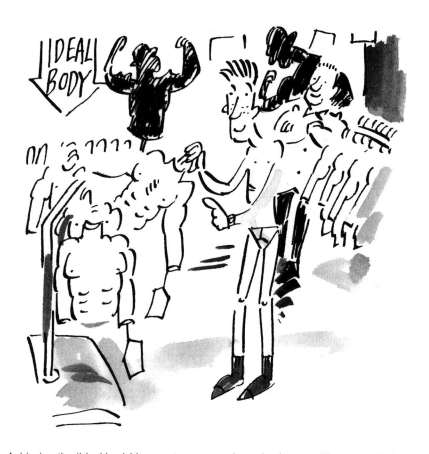

Achieving the 'ideal body' is a contemporary obsession in some Western societies

How do people use their bodies to manage and express a sense of 'identity'?

- Tattooing
- Piercing
- Diet control and manipulation
- Fashion and use of cosmetics
- Fitness regimes
- Cosmetic surgery.

Over to you

- Describe your own body.
- Describe the ways that you use, try to manage or have changed your body to express aspects of your 'self'.

The contemporary use of, and focusing on, the body as a 'site' of social significance has led both sociologists and health-care practitioners to develop new ways of understanding and approaching the human body. This is significant in a variety of areas of health-care practice, given the current associations between 'health', 'illness' and the body.

Understanding the body sociologically

Developing an awareness of the human body as a socially constructed entity can be useful to us in a personal capacity, as well as in our health-carer role. Being aware that we 'read' and understand the human body socially draws attention to the ways that cultural processes, practices and social relations often have an embodied element to them. A sociological understanding of the human body therefore also provides opportunities for us, again in both personal and health-carer capacities, to question, challenge and change some of the oppressive and outdated social constructions of the body that still exist in popular and health-care discourse. This is particularly the case, for example, in relation to expectations of 'able' and 'disabled' bodies as well as sexualised and racialised notions of the body that characterise perceptions of women and members of minority ethnic groups. A sociological understanding of the human body, therefore, provides a basis on which we can rethink and reshape our assumptions about, experiences of and responses to the bodies we have and those of the people we work with.

Thinking about the body

The ways that we perceive, understand and explain the human body reflects the social and cultural beliefs, practices and relations of the historical period in which we live.

Sociological analysis has identified and makes use of a number of different ways of thinking about the human body. First, the human body can be seen as 'real' and 'natural', in essence a biological entity. This is the orthodox approach common within health-care training and practice. Alternatively, the human body can be seen as a social construction. In this sense it gains its meaning within the context of discourses on gender, 'race' and disability, for example. Finally, the human body can be seen and understood in terms of 'lived experience'. This final 'lived body' approach provides something of a link between the 'natural' body approach and the social construction approach.

The 'natural' body

A naturalistic approach to understanding the human body developed in the 18th century with the emergence of medicine as a health-care practice and the growth in power and prominence of 'scientific' thinking. It is now the dominant form of thinking about the body in Western societies generally and in the health-care field in particular.

Because of the overwhelming dominance of the naturalistic approach to the human body, medical meanings of the body now have a **hegemonic** hold over the perceptions and thoughts of many health carers. That is, the power of this naturalistic discourse is so deeply rooted and embedded in our ways of thinking about the human body that it is almost impossible to think of the body as anything other than a 'real', natural, universally common and biologically-based entity.

However, the 'naturalistic' approach to the human body isn't only used to identify and describe its biological basis. The concept of the 'natural' body is also often used to explain a variety of human behaviours and the social relations that can be observed between people. Explanations of 'aggressive behaviour', 'types of personality' and 'temperament', levels of 'intelligence' and forms of 'sexual orientation' are all examples of human behaviours and social differences that are sometimes explained on the basis of a person's 'natural' biological predisposition or embodied essence.

As you would expect, sociological critics reject the claim that the biological basis of the human body can have a direct, determining effect on human social life and relationships. One of the main

● Keywords

Hegemony

An overwhelmingly powerful or politically dominant form of consent given 'spontaneously' by the masses to some form of social arrangement, set of values or ideas.

reasons for this rejection is that so-called 'biologism' neglects the role that culture, social structure and social processes (social context) play in determining individual and collective social experiences and possibilities.

Despite rejecting the biological premise of the naturalistic approach to the human body as reductionist and overly deterministic, some sociological critics still find something interesting and useful in the approach. In particular, they tend to see the naturalistic discourse on the human body as a topic to be studied and explored in itself. This is because the broader use and application of a biological theory of the human body provides us with interesting insights into the existence and use of political ideas and the development of power relations in contemporary society.

The political use of the 'naturalistic' body

The biological 'realities' of the human body have been used to explain and justify a variety of differences and inequalities within the human population. Sociological critics claim that both 'scientific' and common-sense, taken-for-granted discourses contribute to this. The effect, according to these critics, is that the use of 'biology' makes invisible the unequal social and political relations that exist between men and women and dominant and minority ethnic groups, for example.

Men and women *are* biologically different in terms of having differently structured sexual/reproductive organs. However, a naturalistic perspective on the human body has often been employed to justify different work and domestic roles on the basis that differences in the physique of men and women make each more 'naturally' suited to and capable of different types of activity.

Notions of the biologically 'natural' human body are deeply ingrained in all forms of health-care practice. The power of anatomical and physiological representations of the body is rarely challenged or contested by health-care practitioners. However, in pointing out that naturalistic notions of the body are employed in a variety of social and cultural ways, sociological critics of this approach are drawing attention to the political outcomes of representing the body as the source of essential human differences. The idea that a man's distinct biology makes him more suited than a woman to physically demanding work is one example of this. The effect is a socially based division of labour despite the fact that the generalisation does not always hold true. Close reading and analysis of medical textbooks has also shown that male anatomy is often depicted as the 'norm' while female anatomy, by contrast, is presented as deviant (or at best different) from 'the' normal

Stereotypes of …

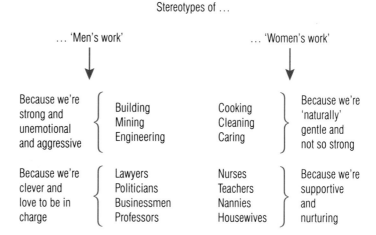

Because we're strong and unemotional and aggressive { Building / Mining / Engineering — Cooking / Cleaning / Caring } Because we're 'naturally' gentle and not so strong

Because we're clever and love to be in charge { Lawyers / Politicians / Businessmen / Professors — Nurses / Teachers / Nannies / Housewives } Because we're supportive and nurturing

Figure 9.1 *Stereotypes of 'men's work' and 'women's work'*

structures (Lawrence and Blixenden 1992). This clearly has implications for the way in which doctors and other health-care practitioners learn about the human body and ascribe meaning to it as they gain their knowledge from textbooks such as this.

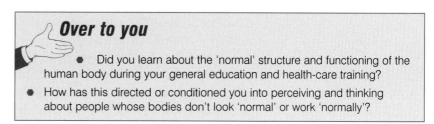

Over to you

● Did you learn about the 'normal' structure and functioning of the human body during your general education and health-care training?

● How has this directed or conditioned you into perceiving and thinking about people whose bodies don't look 'normal' or work 'normally'?

The socially constructed body

The social constructionist approach to the human body is an attempt to challenge the naturalistic perspective and offers a different way of perceiving and relating to the human body. It is an interesting and useful approach for health-care workers who recognise and wish to acknowledge that service users' social and cultural identities are embodied and that protecting and supporting a person's psychological needs and well-being is linked to treating their body with respect and integrity.

There are a variety of forms of social constructionism in relation to the body. Some sociologists, such as Armstrong (1983), argue that the body and disease are the effects or outcomes of discourse (the effect of the 'gaze'). That is, we create the body, or make it visible in a particular way, through the ways that we think about and 'see' it socially and culturally. Others, such as Shilling (1993), argue that the body has a material (biological) base that is shaped and developed by social practices and its social context.

Shilling argues that the body is best thought of as an unfinished biological and social phenomenon. A person can transform their body within changing limits as a result of their participation in society. Shilling's work illustrates how the body is a socially constructed and historically changing entity that is closely linked to our notions of the 'self' and 'identity'. In this sense, the body is a project that we continually work at to accomplish individual self-identity.

Over to you

- Do you have a personal 'body project'?
- What methods are you using to achieve your body project goals?
- To what extent do you think involvement in body projects is 'healthy'? Could it be 'unhealthy'?

If the body is such an important 'site' of social meaning and identity in contemporary society, we need to consider the potential impacts that illness, disability and disease may have on a person's sense of 'self' and identity as well as their physical health and functioning. This awareness that impairment, ill health and disease can have an impact on a person's social and psychological well-being – particularly their self-esteem and self-image – ought to be a part of a health-care worker's knowledge base. Incorporating it into practice is essential if you have a commitment to holistic, person-centred care provision.

The sociological literature on the body and its links to health-care practice also draws our attention to the meaning and impact that a variety of health-care interventions, from surgery to massage and the therapeutic use of touch, may have on a service user's experience of health care and our relationships with service users themselves. Life saving and body-changing technologies operate on both the physical body and social aspects of a person's embodiment. In this sense they may disrupt, as well as enhance or make possible, the 'body projects' of service users. As health-care practitioners it is important for us to be aware that respecting and allowing a person to maintain control over their body is a key way of acknowledging and supporting an individual's sense of autonomy and personal control. Shilling (1993) points out that the body is something that people can have a great deal of control over regardless of the amount of risk and uncertainty that they believe exists in their physical and social environment. Self-control of the body, therefore, is also a means of exerting control over an increasingly complex society. 'Self' and 'identity' then become tied to the body.

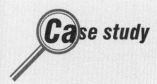

Case study

Chapple, A. and Zieband, S. (2002) Prostate cancer: embodied experience and perceptions of masculinity. *Sociology of Health and Illness*, **24**(6) pp. 820–841.

This study explored the way in which prostate cancer and its treatment affects men's bodies, their roles and their sense of masculinity. Interviews were used to explore the experiences of prostate cancer of 52 men. The study found that existing social constructions of 'masculinity' prevented some men from initially seeking help for prostate-related problems. Treatment tended to affect their sense of masculinity where it had an impact on aspects of bodily functioning such as libido, body shape and energy levels.

Over to you

To what extent can eating disorders such as anorexia nervosa and bulimia nervosa be understood as 'body projects' that reflect both the values and the pressures of living in modern society?

Keywords

Phenomenology

A sociological perspective that argues that sociology should be concerned with everyday surface appearances and not with the hidden depths of society. This involves exploring and analysing things as they are rather than theorising about how we would like them to be. It is therefore very much about everyday knowledge and realities that are experienced.

The 'lived' body approach

A third sociological approach to the body uses a **phenomenological** approach to explore how people use, and construct meaning from using, their bodies to create particular types of social world. The 'lived body' approach focuses on the embodiment of human agency. That is, it focuses on relationships between the self, identity and the body. Sociologists and health-care workers who employ a 'lived body' approach ask questions such as 'How do we use our bodies to act on the world intentionally (expressing agency and constructing identity)?' and 'How do we develop and experience our bodies as part of our sense of "self"?'.

This approach has been used extensively in developing greater understanding of the experience, requirements and potential of people who have chronic health problems or who experience physical or sensory impairment and disability. It is a particularly useful way of enabling and empowering service users who are in this position, and who are typically disempowered and marginalised by 'expert' health-care practitioners, because it privileges 'lived' experience and the views of the service user in the way that their situation and 'needs' are understood. As a result there is a considerable sociological literature on the experience of disability that draws on phenomenological sociology and has contributed significantly to this 'lived body' approach. The following quotation provides a good example of both the importance of listening to 'lived experience' and of the typical neglect of this in care practice situations:

> I've been chronically ill for 12 years. Stroke. Paralysis. That's what I'm dealing with now. I've gone to rehab programme after rehab programme. I may be one of the most rehabilitated people on the face of the earth. I should be President. I've worked with a lot of people. I've seen many types and attitudes. People try very hard to help me do my best on my own. They understand the importance of self-sufficiency and so do I. They're positive and optimistic. I admire them for their perseverance. My body is broke but they still work very hard with it. They're very dedicated. I have nothing but respect for them. But I must say this: I have never, ever, met someone who sees me as a whole. . . .
>
> Can you understand this? Can you? No one sees me and helps me see myself as being complete, as is. No one really sees how that's true at the deepest level. Now I understand that this is what I've got to see for myself, my own wholeness. But when you're talking about what really hurts, and about what I'm really not getting from those who're trying to help me . . . that's it: that feeling of not being seen as a whole.
>
> Dass and Gorman 1986, p. 27

The different perspectives outlined suggest that the human body can be seen as 'natural', 'lived' and 'socially constructed'. Turner (1984) argues that these different approaches to the body can coexist because they focus on different issues and operate at different levels of analysis. As a result, he proposes that we should adopt a pragmatic approach, accepting that the body is naturally (physically) founded while also being socially constructed and 'lived'. Incorporating these sociological insights into your perceptions and understanding of service users' bodies will enable you to avoid the problems associated with impersonal care that is technically efficient while also being disrespectful and damaging to a person's sense of self, autonomy and identity. It is important to be aware that a person's body and the way that you treat it are socially significant.

Caring for the human body

Health-care workers have a particularly unusual relationship with other people's bodies. In an important sense there is now a distinction between a person's 'public body', which they allow others to see and relate to in everyday social situations, and their 'private body', which is unknown to others except in special circumstances. Health-care workers, in appropriate care-related circumstances, appear to occupy a special position in that they are granted rights to breach the public/private distinction that is commonly applied to the body. But how did the public/private distinction develop and what does it involve? The concept of the 'civilised body' can be used to help us to understand this.

The concept of the 'civilised body'

Norbert Elias (1978) argued that the human body has undergone a relatively recent 'civilising process'. He suggested that this process incorporated three progressive processes:

* **Socialisation**: People are encouraged to hide away their natural bodily functions. The body becomes more social than natural and, in fact, some natural functions (vomiting, belching, urinating) come to be evaluated as offensive and distasteful.
* **Rationalisation**: This implies that we are able to control our feelings. We are more rational than emotional.
* **Individualisation**: This highlights the extent to which we see our bodies as encasing and separating our 'selves' from those of others. This is why we maintain a socially acceptable distance from others.

The 'civilised body' is a guarded and regulated, personal body. In many ways this presents problems for health carers who have to work with it, because intimate physical care involves breaching the social boundaries that protect the 'civilised body'. For example, basic physical care often involves touching, seeing and smelling aspects of the human body that are otherwise socially taboo. Nursing care, in particular, is typically about care of the body. As a result it requires practitioners to negotiate the social taboos and boundaries that exist in relation to their patients' bodies. Lawler (1991) identified a variety of ways in which this can be achieved.

Through the creation of a new system of 'rules' in relation to the body: Lawler suggested that the application of four basic rules were necessary for the provision of socially acceptable body care. These include the 'compliance rule', the 'dependency rule' (patients expected to comply with the instructions of the nurse because of their 'dependence' on him/her), the 'modesty rule' (patients expected to avoid being too modest and too embarrassed during body-care routines) and the 'protection rule' (the nurse must acknowledge potential embarrassment and protect patients' privacy).

Through the creation of a set of specific contextors: Lawler suggests that nurses ensure that five 'specific contextors' that 'define the situation' are present when they engage in intimate body care to ensure compliance to these new rules (see above). These 'specific contextors' are:

- Wearing a uniform
- Acting in an appropriate manner
- 'Minifisms'
- Asking relatives to leave before carrying out body care
- Discourse privatisations.

Lawler (1991) found that nurses in her study thought that being 'professional', 'matter-of-fact' and 'in control' were all an important part of body-care situations. Nurses disclosed that they used 'minifisms' by understating or underplaying some events (such as the patient vomiting or being incontinent) in front of the patient. The use of privatisation discourses involved using forms of speech that ensured that certain body functions and aspects of care are kept a private matter between nurse and patient.

Sexuality and genitalia are the most problematic areas of care and conversation in body-care situations. This is particularly the case where gender needs and identities have to be managed as part of the interaction. For example, a body-care situation between a female nurse and a male patient brings into play masculinity and the cultural power of men over women and may involve a level of intimacy not otherwise experienced outside sexual activity. Problems occur when the context of the care situation is disrupted because one of the participants defines the encounter differently.

Over to you

- If you were a patient in hospital unable to meet your physical needs, which aspects of personal or intimate care provision would you most dread?
- What do you think the health-care workers caring for you could do to reduce the worry, embarrassment or stigma of receiving this kind of personal care?

Reflective activity

Reflect on a recent experience of providing or receiving health care in a formal care setting. Apply as many of the sociological concepts and approaches covered in this chapter as you can to your experiences. Reflect on whether they are useful in understanding how notions of 'the body' played a part in and affected your approach to providing or experience of receiving care.

Rapid recap

Check your progress so far by working through each of the following questions.

1. Identify three different ways of thinking about the human body.
2. Explain what sociologists mean when they claim that the body is 'a site of social meaning'.
3. Outline strategies that can be used to make provision of intimate body care for a service user socially acceptable.

If you have difficulty with more than one of the questions, read through the section again to refresh your understanding before moving on.

References

Armstrong, D. (1983) *Political Anatomy of the Body: Medical Knowledge in Britain in the Twentieth Century*. Cambridge University Press, Cambridge.

Dass, R. and Gorman, P. (1986) *How Can I Help? Stories and Reflections on Service*. Alfred A. Knopf, New York.

Elias, N. (1978) *The Civilising Process*, vol 2: *State Formation and Civilisation*. Blackwell, Oxford.

Featherstone, M., Hepworth, M. and Turner, B. S. (eds.) (1991) *The Body: Social Process and Cultural Theory*. Sage, London.

Lawler, J. (1991) *Behind the Screens: Nursing, Somology and the Problems of the Body*. Churchill Livingstone, Edinburgh.

Lawrence, S.C. and Blixenden, K. (1992) His and hers: male and female anatomy in anatomy texts for US medical students 1890–1989. *Social Science and Medicine*, **35**, 925–934.

Shilling, C. (1993) *The Body and Social Theory*. Sage, London.

Turner, B. S. (1984) *The Body and Society*. Blackwell, Oxford.

Further reading

Turner, B. S. (1994) *Regulating Bodies: Essays in Medical Sociology*. Routledge, London.

Sociological approaches to mental distress

Learning outcomes

By the end of this chapter you should be able to:

- Describe the main ideas, assumptions and criticisms of medical psychiatry

- Discuss the strengths and weaknesses of the anti-psychiatry critique of medical approaches to 'mental illness'

- Outline ways of applying sociological concepts and findings to mental health issues that arise in health-care practice.

Approaches to mental distress

Sociological overviews of this topic area tend to begin with the notion that concepts and definitions of mental 'health' and 'illness' should be disputed and contested. In particular, there is a long tradition within the sociological community of contesting whether 'mental illness' is a reality and of disputing the causes of mental distress. In the following sections we will consider how 'mental health' and 'mental illness' are defined by various interest groups. These include health-care practitioners using a traditional medical model approach as well as care practitioners who reject this in favour of 'anti-psychiatry' and other psychosocial approaches to mental distress.

People tend to take a particular position or have a specific perspective on mental distress because of the type of interest or stake that they have in relation to mental health issues – as an individual, service user, relative, doctor, nurse or alternative health practitioner, for example. As a result, people have various ways of understanding mental health issues and respond to the experience of mental 'distress' (their own and that of others) in diverse ways.

Over to you

What are the words, phrases and images that you associate with 'mental health' as an area of health-care practice?

Psychiatry and the medical model

As in a number of other areas of health and illness, sociological approaches to mental distress tend to begin with a critique of the orthodox, dominant medical psychiatry approach to mental distress. Psychiatry provides a set of beliefs and concepts about mental 'health' that are largely based on medical model notions of 'illness' and 'disorder'. These ideas, and the mental health-care practices that result from them, are dominant within the statutory mental health system in the UK and in developed, westernised countries generally.

Medically qualified psychiatrists tend to believe that mental illnesses originate from biological dysfunction. These include dysfunction of the brain, malfunctioning biochemical processes and the inheritance of 'faulty' genes that predispose people to mental illnesses. Psychiatrists who base their health-care practice on biological psychiatry identify mental illness as being located within the individual who experiences mental 'distress' and exhibits symptoms of behavioural and/or emotional 'disorder'. As such, the more biologically orientated forms of psychiatry tend to underplay, and in more extreme cases ignore, the possible contribution and impact of other non-biological factors (cultural, social, psychological and spiritual, for example) in the causation of mental health problems.

Understanding psychiatric diagnosis

The psychiatric diagnosis of 'mental illness' follows a slightly different process from medical diagnosis of physical health problems. Practitioners of both psychiatric and physical medicine tend to look for evidence of 'abnormality' within an individual. However, where

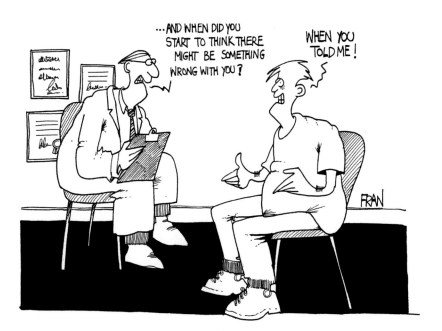

(From Open University course K257 Module 1, The Contested Nature of Mental Health)

practitioners of physical medicine carry out tests and can see clinical 'signs' of physical 'abnormality' (high blood pressure, unusual pulse rates, 'abnormal' biochemistry results, bruising, fractures and bleeding, for example), psychiatrists can't directly see mental 'abnormality'. The 'mind', unlike the physical organs of the body, can't be located or directly observed. As a result, psychiatric practitioners look for patterns of behaviour and emotional 'symptoms' (low mood, poor sleep, loss of appetite, lack of energy) to diagnose 'mental illness' (such as 'depression'). In particular combinations, different symptoms are believed to equate to different 'mental illnesses'. A number of mental illness classification systems exist. The International Classification of Diseases (ICD) system is probably the best known and is widely used by psychiatrists in the UK.

The classic response of the psychiatric profession to 'mental illness' is to try to correct the perceived biological imbalance within the individual by prescribing medication or another form of physical treatment, such as electroconvulsive therapy (ECT), for them.

The descriptions of the 'mental illness' model and the diagnostic and treatment approaches of medical psychiatry given here are necessarily generalised. In some ways they stereotype an area of care practice because mental health care incorporates a more diverse range of beliefs, and uses more varied methods of diagnosis and

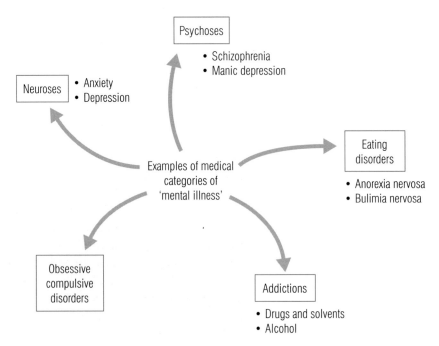

Figure 10.1 *Types of mental illness*

treatment, than this description of medical psychiatry suggests. While I wouldn't deny this, I would argue that the psychiatric approach to mental distress does not generally acknowledge or incorporate social factors within a list of causes of 'mental illness'. This is one of the main criticisms that sociological critics make of the psychiatric approach to 'mental illness'. However, this is not the only criticism to come out of sociological critique of the psychiatric approach to the mental health field generally.

Challenges to psychiatric knowledge and control

Over to you

Look at the following patient 'presentations':

- A stressed, anxious mother of three children under 5 who complains of 'feeling inadequate and useless'.
- A teenager who cannot sleep without taking a sedative tablet.
- A teacher who is losing control over his alcohol consumption as a new term approaches.
- A truanting and 'glue-sniffing' schoolchild who is out of her parents' control.
- A newly married woman who is fearful of sex and is unable to tell her husband.
- An older woman with a failing memory and failing ability to concentrate.
- A man who regularly visits his GP with vague symptoms or minor complaints that have no physical symptoms.
- A business woman who experiences incapacitating headaches when faced by extra pressure at work.

Are any or all of these people 'mentally ill'? Whatever you decide, reflect on how you made your decision about each person.

Each of the people referred to in the above activity seems to have problems with living, coping and establishing a sense of psychological and emotional 'well-being'. While they may share many of the characteristics and experiences of the 'mentally healthy', their problems, and the distress they experience as a result of them, differentiate them both from their 'normal selves' and from other, apparently mentally 'healthy', people. This comparison with a 'normal' self and with others is often important in identifying mental illness. It may well be that each of these individuals is experiencing some mental distress at this point in their life. However, in order to establish a clinical diagnosis you would need to be aware of and identify a particular, characteristic pattern of clinical signs and symptoms in their presentation.

Sociological critics of psychiatry challenge the medical claim that the experience of mental distress is primarily the result of 'illness' and that it is caused by factors within the individual experiencing it. Despite being sceptical, sociological critics of psychiatric knowledge don't necessarily adopt the same approach to these issues. Some critics, typically those adopting an interactionist approach, fundamentally dispute the reality of 'mental illness'. That is, they contest the psychiatric claim that behaviour identified as 'mental illness' is fundamentally different from other forms of behaviour. Instead, they tend to investigate reasons why certain forms of behaviour come to be viewed as 'mental illness' and why some people (rather than others) are labelled as 'mentally ill'.

Is 'mental illness' a myth?

Thomas Szasz (1961) contested the claim that physical and mental illness are similar phenomena. Despite being a psychiatrist himself, Szasz argued that the term 'mental illness' is an inappropriate description of the mental distress that people experience. In fact, Szasz went as far as to argue that 'mental illness' didn't really exist. Instead, Szasz viewed 'mental illness' as a socially constructed myth maintained by the psychiatric profession. This is a controversial claim, given the widespread use and acceptance of psychiatric definitions of 'mental illness'.

Szasz's claim that 'mental illness' is a myth was based on an acceptance of the argument that diagnosis of physical 'illness' is based on objective knowledge of biological, physiological and anatomical dysfunction or abnormality deviating from a normal healthy state. He then argues that 'mental illness', by contrast, cannot be diagnosed or described in similar terms because the 'mind' is not located like an organ within the body. Knowledge of human biology, anatomy and physiology therefore doesn't provide any special insight into the workings of the human mind. Mental 'distress' is therefore not the result of 'disease' in the conventional medical sense.

What is mental 'distress' if it's not 'illness'?

Szasz (1971) argued that people who are diagnosed as suffering from 'mental illness' are really experiencing 'problems in living'. These are essentially social problems, not biomedical problems. Szasz saw 'mental illness' as a metaphor, not a 'fact'. He saw it as a way of dealing with people whose behaviour, beliefs and thoughts 'violate certain ethical, political and social norms' (Szasz 1974,

p. 23). As a result, Szasz (1974) saw the institutional, organised forms of psychiatric care as being repressive, coercive and performing a social control function in modern society. He argued that the role of the psychiatrist was to impose and police socially acceptable 'reality'. People who didn't accept, fit in with or exhibit conventional or acceptable forms of thinking, behaving and perceiving reality were, in Szasz's terms, deprived of their liberty and human right to self-determination by psychiatry.

The anti-psychiatry critique of 'mental illness'

Along with Thomas Szasz, Ronald Laing (1967) was a well-known figure in the 'anti-psychiatry' movement that developed in the late 1960s and 1970s. Like Szasz, Laing was a psychiatrist who thought and practised in unorthodox ways. He is particularly known for using an 'existential psychology' approach to contest the medicalised psychiatric method of diagnosing and treating 'schizophrenia'. Using this approach, Laing disputed the orthodox psychiatric claim that so-called schizophrenic thoughts and behaviour are 'irrational'. Instead, he argued that it was possible to understand the symptoms and experience of schizophrenia in the context of a person's family dynamics.

Laing (1967) believed that relationships in some families are based on distorted and dysfunctional ways of communicating. Consequently, a confusing and pathological emotional environment can develop that some people will have difficulty coping with. Laing believed that people who faced such problems adopted so-called 'schizophrenic behaviour' as an adaptive reaction to the disturbed family dynamics that they faced. In this way Laing reconceptualised 'schizophrenia' by relocating it outside the person as a response to problematic social relationships and circumstances.

The anti-psychiatry movement, which was heavily influenced by the work of both Thomas Szasz and Ronald Laing, drew on a range of sociological perspectives and concepts to question and redefine our understanding of mental 'health' and 'illness'. This has undoubtedly had a significant effect on thinking within the mental health professions. It has also had an impact on the ways in which both mainstream statutory services and their independent sector counterparts are provided for people who experience mental health problems.

While Thomas Szasz's work was important in drawing attention to the power that psychiatrists possessed, and the potential abuses of human rights that psychiatry could perpetrate, his original and powerful claim that mental illness is a 'myth' has been criticised on a number of grounds. For example, psychiatrists refute the claim that they diagnose mental illness only on the basis of observing people's 'abnormal' social behaviour. They point out that they also look for, and take account of, evidence of psychological disturbance and their patient's own accounts of distress when making their diagnoses. Critics of Szasz have also questioned the way in which he apparently assumes that the 'mind' works separately from the body. Many health-care practitioners now subscribe to the view that the two are linked and that physical disease and illness can lead to mental health problems, and vice versa. Szasz is also criticised for failing to acknowledge the real suffering that mental 'distress' involves for many people and the compassionate and caring responses that psychiatrists and other health-care practitioners within the psychiatric system provide in response to this.

Over to you

How would you identify the difference between a person being 'eccentric' and 'mentally ill'?

Applying sociology to 'mental illness' and distress

So far we've seen that sociological critiques of psychiatry and the medical approach to 'mental illness' have played a significant part in destabilising and casting doubt on the efficacy and effectiveness of conventional psychiatric approaches to 'mental illness'. However, a sceptical sociological approach to the issue of 'mental illness' shouldn't just provide health-care practitioners with critique 'ammunition'. This could be criticised as negative, simply knocking down psychiatry without offering any kind of alternative. As such we should also consider how sociological approaches to mental health problems can be used constructively to understand, support and empower those experiencing mental distress.

Questioning and refusing 'illness' labels

Sociological critics of the notion of 'mental illness' have provided a clear example of the way that sociology can have a powerful influence in the health field. One of the important effects of the sociological critique of 'mental illness' has been to cast doubt on the causes of the mental distress that some people experience. In effect, social interactionism has refocused our attention to consider that at least some of the causes of a person's mental distress may be found externally, in the social world in which they live. This more sociological approach to mental distress also draws our attention to the role that health-care professionals and others play in socially constructing and applying 'mental illness' labels.

Thomas Scheff (1966) is often credited with being the first sociologist to develop a labelling theory of mental illness. Labelling theorists such as Scheff tell us that 'deviance' is relative. That is, they suggest that we should reject the idea that behaviour and beliefs can be defined as either 'normal' or 'deviant' in an objective way. Instead, we should be aware that the behaviours and beliefs that are commonly seen as 'deviant' are, in fact, socially defined. As sociologically alert health-care practitioners we should be aware that service users, their relatives and our colleagues who acquire 'mental illness' labels are not inherently or objectively 'deviant'. They are just thought to be so at a particular time, by people with the power to label them as such, who operate within a particular set of social relations.

An awareness of the social process and relative nature of labelling someone as 'mentally ill' provides us with an opportunity to see past the label and to relate more compassionately to the person behind it. This is important because psychiatric labels that define certain behaviours and beliefs as deviant are particularly 'sticky' and difficult to escape from. Many people with enduring mental health problems become dehumanised and lose their sense of individuality and identity as a result of their diagnostic label becoming a master status. Health-care practitioners who accept and apply psychiatric labels are therefore in danger of policing the boundaries of 'normality' rather than practising an objective, value-free form of health care.

Sociological critics who adopt a labelling approach to 'mental illness' see 'deviant' labels as being the product of social interactions in which those who create and maintain 'mental illness' labels do so by applying greater social power over those being labelled. Clearly, health-care practitioners who seek to acknowledge and accept a person's self-defined identity, beliefs and individuality should not unquestioningly accept 'mental illness' labels or diagnoses as providing adequate insight into the person they are caring for. In the end, judging whether a behaviour or belief is 'deviant' is, following interactionism, a moral one. In this sense, positive mental health care should be about identifying and working towards meeting the needs of the individual rather than about responding to medically defined diagnostic labels.

The social distribution of 'mental illness'

Health-care practitioners and academics who adopt structuralist approaches to mental health problems typically seek to identify how mental illness is distributed throughout society. In doing so they tend to accept dominant medical definitions of 'mental illness'. This is often because official government statistics on mental health issues are compiled from doctors' records of psychiatric consultations and patients' contact with medically based mental health services.

Structuralist approaches to 'mental illness' are useful to health-care practitioners, despite the reservations we may have about defining 'mental illness', because they give some insight into how such problems are socially distributed. This, in itself, provides a basis on which to question the idea that mental health problems do not discriminate between people and can strike randomly. Statistics on the social distribution of mental health problems suggest that in fact the contrary is true. Some social groups are more likely to experience mental health problems than others. Additionally, this kind of data also provides a basis on which to argue that many of the causes of mental health problems are external to the individual and are social rather than biological in nature (see Smail 1993 for an interesting account of this).

Using a structuralist approach it is possible to examine the relationship between aspects of social structure such as social class, gender and 'race' or ethnicity and the incidence and prevalence of 'mental illness' in society. Sociologically it is then possible to argue that there are links between environmental stresses, socioeconomic circumstances, social pressures and the occurrence of mental distress. Mental health practitioners who subscribe to a social psychiatry model tend to use this kind of sociological approach to inform their practice.

The social patterning of 'mental illness'

How prevalent is 'mental illness' in society? What is its specific incidence within, and distribution across, different social groupings? Epidemiological data on the prevalence of psychiatric morbidity in the population of the UK reveal how commonly symptoms of mental ill health are experienced and give some insight into the differing patterns of prevalence between social groups in the population. Figures 10.2 and 10.3 describe the relative prevalence of various kinds of mental morbidity by gender.

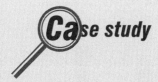

The social causes of depression

A classic sociological study that adopted a structural approach to the causes of mental illness linked the experience of life events and social class position to the occurrence of depression. Brown and Harris (1981) identified social class differences in the distribution of depression. In particular, working-class women with children living at home were more likely than middle-class women or their childless working-class counterparts to develop depression. They were most likely to develop depression if they experienced a significant life event when they were also exposed to:

● Lack of employment outside the home

● Having three or more children under 15 living at home

● Lack of an intimate, confiding relationship with a husband or boyfriend

● Loss of mother before 11 years of age.

The above factors were seen to perform a protective function. As such, a sociological study identified social support as a key factor in protecting people from depression. This insight informs the practice of many professional mental health workers as well as the activities of informal support groups and the approach many of us take to personal relationships.

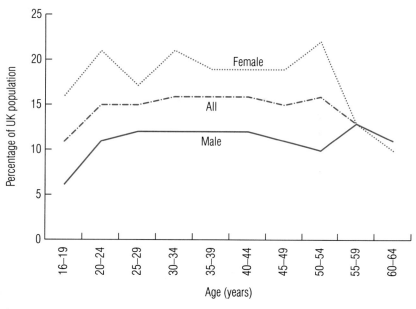

Figure 10.2 *Mental illness by age and sex (from Mind 2000)*

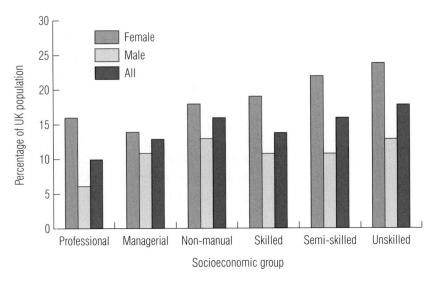

Figure 10.3 *Adults in Britain with significant mental health problems, by socioeconomic group (from Mind, 2000)*

Social class and mental illness

Social class patterns of mental illness reveal high rates among the lower social classes. This is particularly the case for psychoses, such as schizophrenia. This finding is replicated in cross-cultural comparative studies. In contrast, the incidence of suicide shows no social class gradient. Eating disorders, such as anorexia nervosa, are largely a middle-class (and largely female) phenomenon.

The apparently higher rates of mental illness in lower social classes can be accounted for in a number of ways. First, they may be the result of genetic inheritance. The working-class gene pool may predispose its members more to mental illness than its middle-class counterpart. This explanation depends on the still unproven assumption that mental illnesses have a genetic element to them. A second explanation is that 'mental illness' is evidence of social selection occurring. That is, lower social class may be a consequence of mental illness and not the other way around. People who develop mental illnesses are less able to maintain their socioeconomic position and so drift down the social class scale.

A third explanation is that material circumstances, economic disadvantage and a harsher social environment combine to make people in the lower social classes more vulnerable to mental illness than those who live more comfortable, affluent and well-supported lives. Finally, we could also explain the unequal class distribution of mental illness in terms of the differential use of labelling processes. That is, doctors and other psychiatric professionals may have different social expectations of working- and middle-class people in terms of expression and control of behaviour and emotion and use of problem-solving skills. If mental health professionals are mainly middle-class themselves, it is likely that they would hold and apply middle-class norms and values. As such, the higher incidence of working-class 'mental illness' may, in fact, be more indicative of deviation from middle-class norms.

None of the four explanations outlined above provides a complete explanation for the social class gradient in mental illness experience. Sociologists and mental health professionals tend to accept that all play some part in the relationship between mental illness and social class.

Gender and mental illness

According to hospital admission and GP contact data, as well as self-report surveys, women are more likely to experience mental illness than men. This is particularly the case for mood-related disorders, so-called 'personality disorder' and rates of attempted suicide. The data suggest similar levels of experience of psychoses.

Interpreting the statistical evidence is a controversial process. Many argue that the higher rates of mental illness recorded for women are a consequence of different patterns of diagnosis resulting from differing social expectations of men and women. In some ways, diagnoses are 'gendered'. Additionally, it is possible that gender socialisation makes it more likely that women are able to identify, talk about and reveal their psychological and emotional problems than men. The cultural expectations we have of men may therefore act as a barrier to them revealing the real extent of their mental health problems. Therefore, the 'true' incidence of mental illness could be both under- and over-reported for the different genders.

Possible explanations for the gender differences in the incidence of mental illness include:

- Biological explanations such as the effects of hormones
- Social causation explanations such as structural positioning, poverty, maternal deprivation, social isolation, social stress and power differences
- Labelling explanations such as sex stereotypes informing diagnosis.

In practice, the causes of women's mental health problems are likely to encompass all the above and will depend on specific, individual circumstances.

Ethnicity and mental illness

The main problem in this area is defining 'ethnicity' (see p. 79 for more on this). Both 'official' and self-defined definitions of ethnicity have been used to survey the incidence of mental illness in the minority ethnic population. Both have their problems and limitations. The findings of such surveys are complex and often contradictory. For example, Nazroo (1997) conducted a national survey of British ethnic minorities and found that British people of African–Caribbean origin are more likely to experience depression than the majority of the population. He found that their rates of other forms of mental illness were broadly similar to the majority population. However, Koffman *et al.* (1997) found that people of African–Caribbean background were over-represented in treatment for psychotic disorders compared to the majority population. Suman Fernando (2003), a psychiatrist and writer, argues that this latter pattern of over-representation is a reflection of a cultural bias in Western psychiatry rather than any evidence of higher rates of mental illness in the African–Caribbean community.

While explanations for these patterns of mental illness experience tend to follow those for social class and gender, it is also clear that the effects of discrimination, labelling and the social stress caused by racism also have to be taken into account in any analysis of them.

Characteristics of people at high risk of developing mental health problems (Wise 1997)

Adults who are:

- Undergoing divorce or separation
- Unemployed
- At risk of depression in pregnancy
- Experiencing bereavement
- Long-term carers of people who are highly dependent.

Children who are:

- Living in poverty
- Showing behavioural difficulties
- Experiencing parental separation and divorce
- Within families experiencing bereavement.

Reaching a sociological compromise

Sociologists who accept the validity of medical definitions of 'mental illness' tend to argue that the origins and development of mental illnesses are due to a variety of factors. Typically, these include biological factors such as predisposing genes and faulty brain biochemistry, social factors such as stressful life events and oppressive social circumstances and psychological factors such as negative thinking strategies and poor coping skills. This kind of approach incorporates sociological factors into an explanation of the causes of mental illness in a way that is acceptable to, and can be used by, multidisciplinary teams of mental health workers.

The stress–vulnerability model of mental illness (Figure 10.4) provides a way of locating the occurrence of mental illness within a social context and sphere of social relations without saying that these structural and relational features of society are directly responsible for mental illness occurring. Instead they are seen to

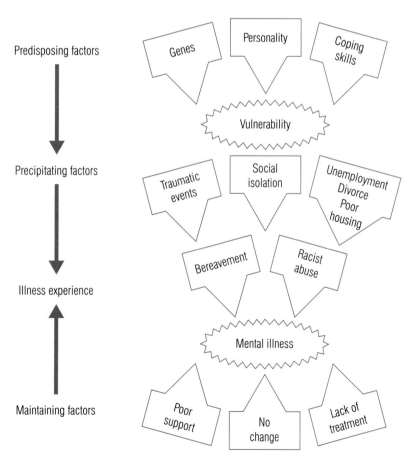

Figure 10.4 *The stress–vulnerability model of mental illness causation*

play a part in the causality of mental illness. This does not question the reality of dysfunction occurring at a biological level or suggest that mental illness is a socially constructed myth.

Reflective activity

Reflect on the sociological critiques of medical psychiatry that you have read about in this chapter. To what extent do you think they can help to reduce fear of 'mental illness' and normalise the experience of mental distress?

Rapid recap

Check your progress so far by working through each of the following questions.

1. Identify two ways in which conventional psychiatric notions of 'mental illness' are contested sociologically.
2. What social factors might account for gendered patterns of mental morbidity?
3. How does the stress–vulnerability model of mental illness use social factors to account for the occurrence of mental illness?

If you have difficulty with more than one of the questions, read through the section again to refresh your understanding.

References

Brown, G. W. and Harris, T. O. (1981) *Social Origins of Depression: a Study of Psychiatric Disorder in Women*. Tavistock, London.

Fernando, S. (2003) *Cultural Diversity, Mental Health and Psychiatry: The Struggle Against Racism*. Brunner-Routledge, London.

Koffman, J., Fulop, N. J. and Pashley, D. (1997) Ethnicity and use of acute psychiatric beds: one-day survey in North and South Thames Regions. *British Journal of Psychiatry*, **171**, 238–241.

Laing, R. D. (1967) *The Politics of Experience*. Penguin, Harmondsworth.

Mind (2000) Mental health statistics: how common is mental distress? Mind Factsheet. Mind, London.

Nazroo, J. Y. (1997) *The Health of Britain's Ethnic Minorities*. Policy Studies Institute, London.

Scheff, T. J. (1966) *Being Mentally Ill: A Sociological Theory*. Aldine Press, Chicago.

Smail, D. (1993) *The Origins of Unhappiness: A New Understanding of Personal Distress*. HarperCollins, London.

Szasz, T. (1961) *The Myth of Mental Illness*. Routledge & Kegan Paul, London.

Szasz, T. (1971) *The Manufacture of Madness*. Routledge & Kegan Paul, London.

Szasz, T. (1974) *Ideology and Insanity*. Penguin, Harmondsworth.

Wise, J. (1997) Health professionals can prevent mental health problems. *British Medical Journal*, **315**, 327–332.

Further reading

Busfield, J. (1986) *Managing Madness: Changing Ideas and Practice*. Unwin Hyman, London.

Furedi, F. (2003) *Therapy Culture: Cultivating Vulnerability in an Uncertain Age*. Routledge, London.

Heller, T., Reynolds, J., Gomm, R. *et al.* (eds.) (1997) *Mental Health Matters*. Macmillan, Basingstoke.

Pilgrim, D. and Rogers, A. (1994) *A Sociology of Mental Health and Illness*. Open University Press, Buckingham.

Scheff, T. J. (1966) *Being Mentally Ill: A Sociological Theory*. Aldine Press, Chicago, IL.

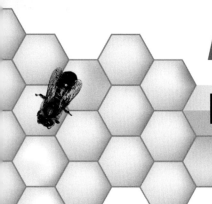

Appendix

Rapid Recap – answers

Chapter 1

1. Identify when and explain why the discipline of sociology first emerged.

1. Sociology emerged in the early 19th century as a response to social upheavals reshaping society during this period.

2. Explain how sociology differs from psychology.

2. Sociology focuses on collective or group issues external to the individual. Psychology tends to focus on internal, individual experiences and processes.

3. Suggest reasons why the 'human-made world' can be seen as a 'social environment'.

3. The 'human-made world' is a social environment because it is constructed or constituted out of social relationships between people and groups at a collective level, because it is socially organised and structured and because people develop and apply social and cultural 'meaning' to make sense of everyday experiences.

Chapter 2

1. What is the difference between 'micro' and 'macro' sociology?

1. Micro sociology focuses on the detail of social behaviour and social processes in society. Macro sociology focuses on the 'big picture' of how society is organised and structured.

2. Identify three features or characteristics of 'sociological thinking'.

2. Sociological thinking is characterised by a sceptical, questioning and critical approach to 'taken-for-granted' assumptions, by a focus on the 'social' aspects of health at a micro and macro level, and by the way that 'individualist' explanations are contested.

3. Explain why sociological thinkers tend to reject individualist explanations of health and illness experience.

3. Sociological thinkers tend to reject individualist explanations of health and illness experience because these approaches ignore the role and impact of broader social structures and processes and because they are seen as blaming particular groups of people for their 'failure' or 'inadequacies'.

Chapter 3

1. Identify two ways of approaching health-care issues sociologically.

1. Positivistic (scientific) and naturalistic (interpretive) approaches.

2. Explain the difference between a social structure and a social action focus within sociology.

2. A social structure approach focuses on the macro or 'big picture' issues and will tend to be positivistic. A social action approach focuses on the micro level of social experience and social processes using a naturalistic approach.

3. Describe the main concerns of feminist and anti-racist standpoint perspectives within sociology.

3. Feminist perspectives examine the social world from the standpoint of women, considering issues and factors that have a particular impact on women's lives. Anti-racist perspectives examine the social world from the standpoint of marginalised

black and minority ethnic (BME) groups, considering issues and factors that cause and perpetuate racial prejudice and unfair discrimination.

Chapter 4

1. Identify when and describe why the biomedical model of health care emerged.

1. The biomedical model of health care emerged in the 18th century as 'science' usurped religion as the key system of knowledge and 'truth' about 'health'.

2. Outline three ways in which sociological critics have challenged the biomedical model of the medical profession.

2. Sociological critics have claimed that individualised medical knowledge neglects the social context and broad social patterning of disease and illness experience, that it socially constructs' ideas of 'disease' and 'illness', leading to the medicalisation of social life, and that medical knowledge and practice operates as a form of social control in modern society.

3. Identify and describe two alternative approaches to the biomedical model of health care.

3. Public health medicine uses an alternative 'social' approach to disease and illness experience. Alternative or complementary therapies offer different ways of thinking about 'health' and the factors that affect it.

Chapter 5

1. Define the terms morbidity, mortality and standardised mortality rate.

1. Morbidity refers to illness. Mortality refers to death. The standardised mortality rate refers to 'average' death rates for defined groups of people.

2. Describe three ways of conceptualising Britain's social class structure.

2. Britain's social class structure can be thought of as a three-class 'pyramid', as a more differentiated, multiclass 'pyramid' (Registrar General's scale) or as a diamond-shaped structure (NS-SEC scale).

3. Outline the key finding of sociological studies into the link between social class and health experience and identify four explanations for it.

3. The key finding is that mortality rates follow a social class pattern – people in the higher social classes live longer than people in the lower social classes. This may be explained as an artefact of research, as an effect of social selection, as a consequence of cultural behaviours or as the result of structural forces having greater impact on lower social classes.

Chapter 6

1. Define the terms 'sex' and 'gender'.

1. 'Sex' refers to the biological definition of a person as either 'male' or 'female'. 'Gender' refers to the cultural and social attributes and expectations of men and women in society.

2. Why, according to sociologists, is it important to distinguish between sex and gender when exploring women's health issues?

2. Sociologists distinguish between sex and gender to identify how expectations of men and women are constructed socially and politically in 'gender' terms and to explore the impact that 'gender' has on social opportunities and experiences.

3. Describe the ways in which patterns of morbidity and mortality are 'gendered' and outline how these gender patterns can be explained.

3. Women report more ill-health but have lower premature mortality rates and greater life expectancy than men. Explanations focus on 'artefact', genetic factors, structural forces and culture/lifestyle as possible influences on this.

Chapter 7

1. Explain why the concept of 'race' is contested and usually rejected by sociologists.

1. 'Race' is contested because it is seen as a social construction that is a product of value judgements about the supremacy of 'white' people.

2. **Define the term 'racism' and explain how 'racial discrimination' is said to involve more than 'bad behaviour' by individuals.**

2. Racism is prejudice and unfair discrimination against members of another ethnic group. Racial discrimination is alleged to involve institutional and societal assumptions, arrangements and processes that privilege or favour some ethnic groups to the disadvantage of others.

3. **Outline three contrasting explanations for the ethnic patterning of health and illness experience in Britain.**

3. Contrasting explanations include those based on biological/genetic theories, structural explanations, culture and lifestyle and artefact explanations.

Chapter 8

1. **Identify three popular ways of explaining the causes of 'illness'.**

1. Popular explanations of illness distinguish between 'normal' and 'real' illness, see it as an 'invasion' of germs, as bodily 'degeneration' or 'damage' and as 'imbalance'.

2. **Describe what happens during the 'social process' of becoming ill.**

2. The social process of becoming ill involves the lay recognition and then 'official' confirmation of physical or mental experiences as 'illness'.

3. **Explain how the concepts of 'deviance', 'labelling' and 'stigma' can be used to understand social responses to certain forms of 'illness'.**

3. Deviance, labelling and stigma are used to explain how certain 'illness' behaviours attract social disapproval and sanctions because they depart from cultural norms and expectations.

Chapter 9

1. **Identify three different ways of thinking about the human body.**

1. The 'natural' body, the 'socially constructed' body and the 'lived body'.

2. **Explain what sociologists mean when they claim that the body is 'a site of social meaning'.**

2. The notion of the body as a site of social meaning refers to the idea that people invest social meaning in the way that they use and experience their own and other people's bodies, particularly through applying discourses of 'race', 'gender' and 'disability' to the body.

3. **Outline strategies that can be used to make provision of intimate body care for a service user socially acceptable.**

3. Provision of socially acceptable body care is achieved through applying the rules of 'compliance', 'dependency', 'modesty' and 'protection' and through the use of 'specific contextors' (see Lawler 1991, in text).

1. **Identify two ways in which conventional psychiatric notions of 'mental illness' are contested sociologically.**

1. Sociologists contest the notion that the causes of mental distress are located within the individual. Some sociologists offer a more radical critique by disputing the validity of 'mental illness', claiming that it is a socially constructed myth.

2. **What social factors might account for gendered patterns of mental morbidity?**

2. Gendered patterns of diagnosis may be the result of gender stereotypes and assumptions. Alternatively, women may reveal and talk about their experiences of mental distress more readily than men, thereby increasing opportunities for diagnosis and treatment. Other possible explanations include biological differences and labelling processes.

3. **How does the stress-vulnerability model of mental illness use social factors to account for the occurrence of mental illness?**

3. The stress vulnerability model sees social factors as precipitating and maintaining the predisposition that people have towards mental illness.

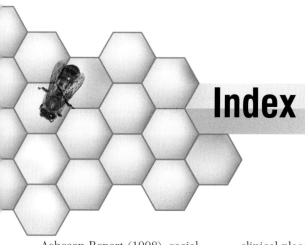

Index